THE NEW FORMAT

GRE

TEST PREP BOOK

2025 – 2026

The Ultimate Guide to Ace the GRE on Your First Attempt with Real Practice Tests

299+ practice problems

Exampro 365

This book is published by ExamPro 365 Publishers.

Kindle Editon: 978-1-965849-43-9

Paperback Edition: 978-1-965849-44-6

First Edition: 2025

Printed in The USA

Table of Contents

INTRODUCTION

Are you tired of sifting through half-baked GRE prep materials that promise the world but leave you confused, overwhelmed, and second-guessing your every move? Are you done with stuffy lectures that drone on about formulas or vocabulary words you'll never actually use? Then brace yourself. You're holding the single most ruthless, results-driven GRE resource on the market—an unflinching, high-octane arsenal designed to blast through the test writers' traps and lead you straight to victory.

Welcome to a book that refuses to pamper you with hollow reassurances or lofty academic jargon. This is a no-nonsense, hard-hitting GRE companion built for the serious contender who wants to crush the exam on the first go. Don't believe me? The countless success stories from real people who've used this guide—and walked away with results that catapulted them into top graduate programs—should get your attention. Let's hear a few of these reviews:

1. **Jessica P., 330 scorer, Georgetown University-bound:**

"I was drowning in a sea of conflicting resources—flashcards here, random online quizzes there—until I grabbed this book. The strategies aren't gentle suggestions; they're step-by-step instructions designed to tear the exam apart. My score shot up by over 12 points in a month, and I owe every bit of that improvement to the brutal honesty and powerful tactics inside these pages."

2. **Aiden R., 335 scorer, from a small liberal arts school:**

"People told me, 'You need a fancy tutor or a big-name prep class if you're serious.' I couldn't afford that. This book gave me everything—timing strategies, mental frameworks, next-level reading comprehension tips. There's no fluff. It's direct, it's intense, and guess what? I blew through the GRE's hardest questions like they were baby puzzles."

3. **Monica F., scored 170 Quant, 164 Verbal, scholarship winner:**

"I've never been a math genius, but the quant sections in this book are unbelievably clear and cutthroat. Not only did I learn how to solve the problems, but I also learned how to dominate the clock, guess smartly, and exploit the test's vulnerabilities. My GRE success unlocked a scholarship, and that scholarship changed my life."

These aren't polite endorsements you'd find sprinkled in casual marketing blurbs. These are the battle cries of victors—real test-takers who stepped onto the GRE battlefield armed with this single resource, hammered through the challenges, and walked away with the spoils. And now, you're next in line.

Let's make one thing crystal clear: The GRE is not your friend. It's a gatekeeper, an elaborate puzzle specifically engineered to stress you out and pick apart your weaknesses. It has entire armies of question types—Text Completion, Reading Comprehension, Data Interpretation sets, geometry nightmares—lined up to exploit any ignorance or poor time management you bring to the table. Most books tiptoe around this reality, offering you bland and 'safe' advice that feels good but lacks teeth. They'll say, "Pace yourself wisely," or "Memorize these 500 words." Not here. Here, you'll get the real story of how the GRE tries to get in your head, how it manipulates your sense of timing, and how you can systematically disarm every trap.

From page one to the final practice question, this book is a call to arms. You will learn to read the test's mind, anticipate which corners they cut in question design, and harness that inside knowledge to your advantage. Every single topic—from those dreaded triple-blank Text Completions to the often-misunderstood experimental section—will be dissected with surgical precision. We'll show you exactly where the GRE math can be twisted or simplified so you have a map to avoid the common pitfalls. You'll discover advanced reading techniques that slash through the fluff of reading passages and reveal the only lines you need to focus on. This methodology doesn't rely on luck or natural brilliance; it's the product of hardcore analysis, daily practice, and feedback from test-takers just like you.

Of course, none of this matters if you aren't committed to the program. This is not a half-measure or a quick fix. Reading a single chapter and giving up won't magically net you that 330+ score. You have to commit to the intensity. The chapters you're about to read demand your sweat: you'll be charting your mistakes, analyzing your guesses, identifying your pacing flaws, and hammering them out until they're gone. If you've got a thin skin for accountability, you might balk. But if you're serious about commanding your future—if you want to walk into the test center feeling like you've already conquered the exam in practice—then you're in the right place.

Let's talk about motivation. People often approach the GRE like it's just an annoying chore: "It's something I have to do so I can apply to grad school." That's a dangerous mindset because it invites you to just 'get through it' rather than excel. You need a stronger, sharper outlook: "This test can open or lock the doors to my future. I'm going to crush it." There's nothing moderate about success in these competitive times. A half-baked approach to GRE prep is the fastest path to rejections and regrets. This resource will ignite a fire under you, waking you up to the fact that a strong GRE score can be the difference between a fully funded dream school and a polite rejection letter.

And that's why we won't hesitate to push you hard. With a test as critical as the GRE, you can't afford to tiptoe around. Each chapter in this guide is designed not just to teach, but to transform. You'll be challenged to break your own patterns, unlearn old study habits that do nothing but waste time, and adopt an ultra-focused system that has proven itself, time and again, for every type of learner. Whether you're a quick study or you struggle with test anxiety, the blueprint here will force you to measure your progress in real terms—by actual scores, timed sections, and practical mastery, rather than warm, fuzzy feelings.

Still skeptical? Listen to a few more voices from people who once stood where you are now:

- **Leon R., struggling math student turned 168 Quant achiever:**

"I hated math my whole life. Thought I was doomed to guess my way through the GRE. Then I found the step-by-step breakdowns in this book—complete with advanced shortcuts for geometry, data analysis, and algebra. The style is so direct it felt almost militaristic, but it worked. My final quant score was 168, and my acceptance letters started rolling in."

- **Priya K., overcame test anxiety to secure a 327 total:**

"I would freeze up during practice tests, losing precious time. I came across the psychological hacks in this guide—specific breathing patterns, pacing tactics, mental reframes. They're spelled out like a mission plan. I implemented them, and my nightmares about the GRE basically disappeared. I went from panic to power mode."

These words aren't hype—they're a glimpse into how unstoppable you can become with the right tools. The plain fact is that you don't need three different prep courses or a million flashcards if you follow this guide religiously. This single resource has everything you need, from the granular mastery of content to the high-level strategies that blow past common mistakes. There's no filler, no babble, no contradictory tips. It's lean, focused, and hungry for results—just like you should be.

So consider this your official wake-up call. Stop playing nice with your future. Stop fiddling around with a thousand free resources that spread you thin. Dive into this manual with both eyes open and commit to the techniques you're about to discover. Each chapter is your training ground; each practice set is your arena. And when you finally walk into the test center, you won't be crossing your fingers for luck. You'll already be in attack mode—ready, armed, and fully confident in your ability to outsmart any question the GRE dares throw at you.

If you're still comfortable with average results, you can set this book aside. But if you're ready to rampage through mediocrity and forge a new path—one that ends with you sporting an unassailable GRE score—turn the page. Strap in. Follow the plan. Own your future.

Because once you commit to this resource, there's no turning back. This is the only GRE guide that will systematically knock down every barrier standing between you and the graduate school acceptance letter of your dreams. It's not safe, it's not soft, and it sure isn't gentle—but if you're ready for success, it will be your greatest ally.

Welcome to the battle. Let's crush the GRE toaether.

CHAPTER 1: Conquer the Clock and Exploit Every Question

This is your battle cry: The GRE will not wait for you. Time is your single greatest enemy on test day, and you must dominate it to emerge victorious. The test-makers have set the clock ticking, and every passing second wants to sabotage your calm, your strategy, and your focus. This chapter gives you a concrete, battle-tested plan to ensure that the clock works *for* you—not against you. It also shows you how to turn "guessing" from a desperate, random hail-mary into a methodical approach that rescues critical points. By the time you finish reading, you'll know exactly how to pace yourself, guess effectively, and channel your energy toward the exact question in front of you—no matter how tough it looks.

Time Is Your Greatest Enemy

Pace Yourself Wearing a watch is non-negotiable. Yes, many testing centers offer on-screen timers, but they're easy to overlook in the pressure cooker that is the GRE. Your own watch keeps you grounded: it's your personal scoreboard telling you where you stand at every turn. The moment the test begins, check the time. Note how many minutes you have for the section. Then, after every few questions, glance at your watch to see if you are behind, right on schedule, or ahead of pace.

- **The Rushed Trap**

  Eventually, you might find yourself forced to speed up. *Don't panic.* Resist the urge to scramble in a blind guessing spree. Instead, accelerate smartly. Quickly eliminate answers you suspect (or know) are wrong. If you're running exactly one minute behind, there is no reason to skip an entire question or throw random guesses for the next three. Instead, for the *next four* questions, shave off about 15 seconds each—just enough time to catch back up. Once you recover your time, return to your normal pace, focusing on accuracy.

- **Let It Go**

  After you've made a hurried guess on a difficult question, don't keep mentally circling back and agonizing over it. If it was that time-consuming, it was probably a tough or ambiguous question. You are *likeliest* to miss the hardest questions anyway, so the guess you made isn't a huge loss. Winning on the GRE is about maximizing your total correct answers, not flawlessly analyzing one monstrous question.

- **When You're Ahead**

Surprising as it may sound, if you find yourself well ahead of schedule, it might help to *slow down*. Double-check tricky details. The GRE punishes careless mistakes, and finishing 10 minutes early only to have missed easy points is the definition of heartbreak. High-scoring test-takers often have time left over, so their biggest threat can be rushing unnecessarily. Slow down, watch for hidden traps, and maintain a calm, careful pace.

Why the Clock Matters

To excel, you need a mental framework that says: *I will always know how far ahead or behind I am with my available time.* That awareness keeps you cool under pressure. Forcing yourself to measure your progress in small intervals—maybe every five questions—prevents big, nasty surprises when you suddenly realize you only have five minutes left for 15 problems. You remain the pilot in command, controlling the test rather than letting it control you.

Guessing Is Not Guesswork

You've probably heard that you should guess on the GRE if you're stumped because there's no penalty for a wrong answer. That's 100% true. But do you know *how* to guess for maximum point yield?

The Secret Impact of Proper Guessing Unless you're scoring in the highest stratosphere, guessing will contribute *significantly* to your final score. A random guess at a five-choice question means a 20% chance of being correct. Over the course of multiple questions, that can be a real bump if done *properly*. But guess incorrectly—by letting test-writers trick you into half-baked eliminations—and you might drive your guessing odds *below* 20%. The difference between "random guess" and "uninformed hunch" can be huge.

The Monkey Parable Picture 20 monkeys taking the GRE. Despite having no knowledge or clues, *their* random guesses on stumper questions will net them a consistent 20–25% success rate (depending on the question type). Now imagine 20 real human test-takers: ironically, their guess rate on truly unknown questions might be *less* than 20% because:

1. **Attractive Distractors** – The test-makers cleverly plant answer choices that *look* correct but aren't. A clueless test-taker chooses that enticing trap. By contrast, the monkey's randomness spares it from the test-maker's deviousness.
2. **Faulty Elimination** – Test-takers often eliminate correct answers by "hunches" or "it looks too simple," leaving them with zero chance on that question. Again, the clueless monkey would have kept that correct choice in the running.

The $5 Challenge Here's your remedy: treat every guess as if you're betting *five dollars* on the choice. Before you eliminate a choice, ask yourself, "Would I bet five bucks that this is definitely wrong?" If the answer is no, *don't eliminate it.* This $5 filter curbs the impulsive "guess-and-ditch" decisions that lead to sabotaging your own odds.

1. If you're not $5 sure, keep that choice in the guess pool.
2. If you're $5 sure an option is wrong, eliminate it.
3. If only one or two remain and you're $5 sure, pick the single best guess.

This concept forces you to respect the difference between actual knowledge and a random hunch. It aligns your approach with the real mathematics of probability, ensuring you capture every fraction of a point you can.

Predefined Random Strategy To guarantee your guesses stay *truly* random, decide in advance how you will fill in guesses. One straightforward method: if the $5 test leaves you with multiple choices, *always choose the first among those remaining.* This eliminates your mind's temptation to say, "Oh, but B *looks* better than A." Don't overthink. You maintain consistent, random guesses that preserve the 20% probability when no partial knowledge is available.

Practice Smarter, Not Harder

Many students dread GRE prep because they imagine endless, soul-crushing hours of mindless drilling. That is a recipe for burnout, not for success. The GRE is a complex test that demands not just content knowledge but also strategy, pacing, and endurance. You can't just do *more* practice; you need the *right* practice.

The Mental Marathon Think of the GRE as a mental marathon, not a sprint. Runners don't jump into a 26-mile race after a week's training, and neither should you approach the GRE cold. You have to ramp up systematically:

1. **Get Good Practice Tests**

   Seek out high-quality sources for practice exams. They're essential for diagnosing your problem areas and getting comfortable with real test pacing.

2. **Consider Multiple Guides**

   Different authors have different teaching angles; sometimes an alternative explanation can finally make a stubborn concept click. If you can afford it, cross-reference a couple of good GRE prep books.

3. **Incremental Progress**
    - **Phase 1**: Take a practice test with no time limit and with study aids open. Focus purely on *understanding* every concept and *applying* every strategy.
    - **Phase 2**: Take a practice test with time constraints but keep your aids open. Now you're training your pacing muscles while still reinforcing content.
    - **Phase 3**: Finally, take a test with no open notes and normal time limits. This is your "dress rehearsal."

If you have more time, repeat Phase 3 multiple times with various practice exams. Each cycle refines your technique and conditions your mind to handle the real exam's time pressure.

Prepare, Don't Procrastinate

The test is partly a puzzle, partly a marathon, and partly a reflection of how effectively you can keep your nerves under control. Preparation is your life raft. Never stroll into the official test thinking, "I'll treat this one as practice and take it again." That wasted attempt likely only erodes your confidence. Instead, plan to knock it out on the *first* go:

- Understand the test structure.
- Refine your strategies.
- Sleep well the night before.
- Hit test day with your best shot.

Could you take it multiple times? Sure—but the idea is to minimize the *need* for retakes. Every exam date is precious. If you can nail it once, do so!

Test Yourself

Time is money—yours. So spend it wisely. The *only* way to know you're ready for test day is to take a practice exam that mimics real conditions: real time limits, no aids, no breaks aside from those allowed. If you do extremely well and surpass your goal score, you probably don't need to invest another hundred hours drilling question sets. But if your performance is subpar, get serious. Double down on targeted review of your weaknesses. Keep retesting periodically to benchmark your progress until you break through to your target range.

- **Confidence Through Data**: Walking into your GRE test knowing you've already hit your target score in practice is a massive morale booster. You'll trust your instincts under pressure because they're honed by realistic simulations.

23 test-taking General Strategies

This section distills powerful test-taking tactics that apply to *all* GRE question types. They might sound simple, but each is a proven difference-maker.

1. **Dive In Immediately**

Don't let the GRE's complexity or occasionally strange-sounding terms overwhelm you. Whether it's a geometry proof or a dense reading passage, the best approach is to dive in. Skimming the question passively or fretting about difficulty only wastes time.

2. **Predict the Answer Before Looking at Choices**

For reading comprehension or certain quantitative problems, once you have a sense of what's asked, see if you can articulate *in your own words* what the right answer should say. When you finally look at the official answer choices, you'll have a sharper internal compass pointing you to the correct one.

3. **Answer Only What's Asked**

The GRE is notorious for offering answer choices that are *true* but don't actually *answer* the specific question. Don't pick an answer because it "sounds right" or "makes sense." Confirm that it precisely addresses the question asked.

4. **Benchmark**

When you read the first answer choice, decide if it seems plausible. Temporarily treat it as your "standard," and compare each subsequent choice to that standard. If you find a clearly better choice, that becomes the new standard. This process helps you systematically evaluate each option.

5. **Use All Information**

The GRE doesn't waste question real estate with random fluff. If a question includes two seemingly unrelated details, they *are* related—your job is to figure out how.

6. **Beware Fact Traps**

A fact in an answer choice can be correct but still not address the question. Keep your eyes on the exact wording the GRE uses. "Which of the following best supports the claim above?" is not the same as "Which of the following is true?"

7. **Milk the Question**

If you're stuck, dissect each piece of the question carefully. Replace unfamiliar terms with synonyms if possible, or consider the context. The question might drop subtle hints in the phrasing—especially in adjectives or qualifiers.

8. **Don't Overvalue Familiarity**

GRE test-writers often test your *ability* to handle the unfamiliar. Recognizing a single word in an answer choice can be tempting: "Oh, I know that word—this must be correct!" But if the rest doesn't align with the question, reject it.

9. **Eliminate Wrong Answers**

Cross them out physically (if you have scratch paper) or mentally. Each wrong elimination improves your odds. But remember the $5 principle: only remove an answer if you're truly confident.

10. **Know When to Move On**

If a question is taking too long, do a quick elimination if you can, pick the best guess, and keep going. Don't sacrifice a big chunk of time that could secure multiple correct answers elsewhere.

11. **Brainstorm Methodically**

For tough items, list each possible answer and ask, "Could this answer the question?" Evaluate them in turn. Then choose or guess. Move on.

12. **Read Carefully Yet Efficiently**

It's a balancing act: read thoroughly enough to avoid careless errors, but don't lose yourself in micro-details if the main thread is enough to answer the question.

13. **Stay Grounded**

The GRE seldom demands huge leaps of logic. If an answer choice requires space-time warping or wacky assumptions, it's probably wrong.

14. **Hedge Words**

Pay attention to words like *likely, sometimes, generally, mostly, rarely,* or *often.* They make an answer choice less absolute, which can make it more plausible. Watch out for absolute terms like *always* or *never*—they're rarely correct unless you're absolutely sure.

15. **Switchback Words**

Words like *however, although, nevertheless, despite,* or *on the other hand* signal a change in direction. In reading passages, these pivot words are crucial to the author's argument.

16. **Watch for New Info**

A correct answer typically flows directly from the info given in the question. If an answer choice introduces brand-new concepts or data you can't link to the question, be wary.

17. **Manage Your Time**

Know your pace. If you stumble on an alien concept, skip, guess, or do a partial elimination. Don't let one question wreck your entire section.

18. **Keep Your Cool**

Panicking solves nothing. If your mind goes blank, just start working the problem systematically. Let your training take over.

19. **Answer Selection**

If you find yourself picking a choice too quickly because it "feels right," confirm by checking other options. The GRE loves to dangle credible but incomplete answers.

20. **Double Check**

If time permits, revisit flagged questions or quick guesses. A 30-second review can catch a silly slip that could cost you precious points.

21. **Distrust Exact Duplicate Phrases**

Sometimes an answer choice merely repeats a snippet from the passage or question but doesn't actually solve the question. That's a trap.

22. **Be Skeptical of Extreme Statements**

GRE logic is rarely dogmatic or all-or-nothing. If you see an answer that claims a process "should be discontinued completely," it's probably not the best choice unless your reading explicitly says so.

23. **Opposite or Parallel Answers**

If two or three answer choices are basically the same statement but in opposite directions ("x increases," "x decreases"), the correct answer is often among them. Don't be fooled by an "odd one out" that doesn't match the question's direction.

Top 20 Test-Taking Tips

1. **Follow Registration Procedures**
   Don't wait until the last minute. Missing a registration step can derail months of prep.
2. **Know Test Directions and Format**
   Familiarize yourself with question types, time limits, and the structure of each section.
3. **Set a Study Schedule (3-4 Weeks Minimum)**
   Earlier is better. Plan your daily or weekly tasks so you cover everything.
4. **Study at Your Peak**
   If you're a morning person, set that time for your hardest tasks. Night owls, do the opposite.
5. **Leverage Your Learning Style**
   If you're visual, create mind maps or charts. If auditory, use recordings. Adapt the test content to your strengths.
6. **Focus on Weak Spots**
   It's tempting to keep practicing what you already do well. Attack your weaknesses head-on first.
7. **Team Up**
   A study buddy can keep you accountable and help explain tricky areas.
8. **Practice, Practice, Practice**
   Use timed practice tests. Nothing beats simulating the test-day environment.
9. **Sleep Well**
   No heroic all-nighters. Sleep is crucial to memory and mental performance.

10. **Eat Right**
    Junk food can spike or crash energy. A balanced meal fuels stable focus.
11. **Map Out the Test Site**
    Know how to get there, how long it takes, and where to park. Avoid test-day panic.
12. **Bring Earplugs**
    If the testing center is noisy or you're easily distracted, earplugs can be a lifesaver.
13. **Dress in Layers**
    Testing rooms can be freezing or hot. Layer so you can adapt.
14. **Valid ID**
    Bring at least two current forms of identification. Read your test ticket instructions carefully.
15. **Arrive Early**
    Don't let lateness sabotage your calm. Arrive with time to check in, breathe, and settle.
16. **Eliminate the Obviously Wrong, Then Pick the First Remaining**
    This is your plan for saving time and sticking to a systematic approach.
17. **Pace Yourself**
    If you get stuck, guess and move on. Don't doom your entire test for a single item.
18. **Stay Positive**
    Even if you feel the test is going horribly, stick to your strategy. A meltdown never helps.
19. **Keep Your First Answer**
    Unless you realize an obvious error, your initial instincts are often correct.
20. **Double Check**
    If you have leftover time, recheck your answers—especially the tricky ones.

Mastering your time is the *gateway skill* to GRE success. Every question you answer right or wrong has a time cost. Distribute that time carefully, and remember that your best approach to unknowns is a *methodical guess,* not random hope or tangential elimination. You can pivot from behind-schedule to on-schedule with a few seconds shaved here and there, staying calm and methodical throughout.

Finally, keep your morale high: The GRE can be systematically conquered. It is not a mystical or arbitrary beast. Time and again, test-takers who *own* the clock, who *guess* with intelligence, and who *practice* with discipline come out on top. And that's where you're headed.

Keep reading. Keep drilling. Keep refining. Because while time might be your enemy, you have everything you need to beat the clock—and everything else the GRE throws at you.

CHAPTER 2: 10 Ultimate Building Stamina and Strategy for Total GRE Domination

Time management and guessing strategy might keep you afloat, but if you want to *dominate* the GRE, you'll need deeper preparation methods, unstoppable mental endurance, and an unwavering plan that's immune to test-day jitters. Here, we'll expand on how to integrate your practice regime, how to handle every question type *strategically,* and how to avoid the pitfalls that cost your peers valuable points. We'll also explore how to keep calm, manage stress, and ensure you walk into that exam hall like it's your personal arena.

1. Smarter Practice Redux: Efficiency Over Exhaustion

You've likely heard the phrase "work smarter, not harder." Nowhere is that more critical than on the GRE. You cannot burn yourself out by tackling 1,000 random questions with no targeted approach. Instead, funnel your energy into the areas where it counts:

- **Pinpoint Your Weak Links**

  Maybe geometry is your Achilles' heel, or your reading comprehension falters on lengthy passages. Identify these issues early—through timed diagnostics—and then attack them systematically. Use a multi-phase approach:

1. **Open-Book Drilling:** Zero time constraints, all reference materials allowed. Focus on truly *learning*.
2. **Timed Drilling:** Keep the clock in the background. Still let yourself check references occasionally, but tighten up your pace.
3. **Full Simulation:** No references, strictly timed. Mimic real test conditions.

   Each step builds a different muscle: comprehension, speed, and test-day stamina.

- **"Can I Teach It?" Litmus Test**

A favorite question: If you had to teach a concept (like exponent rules or reading "attitude" questions) to a study partner, *could you?* If not, you don't truly understand it. Teaching forces you to articulate the logic, which cements it in your mind.

- **Intentional Breaks**

You do *not* get extra credit for never stopping your studies. Your brain needs downtime to consolidate new information. Schedule short intervals of rest. Fifteen minutes away from the books can restore your focus for the next hour of practice.

2. Overcoming Procrastination

You've heard it: "I'll start next week" or "I'll just do a quick practice the night before." Procrastination is an invisible anchor dragging down your potential. The solution?

- **Micro Goals**

  Break your big GRE ambition (e.g., "I'll do 10 practice exams!") into smaller, more attainable targets: "This week, I'll master integer properties, do 20 practice problems, and complete two timed essays." Meeting these micro goals is satisfying, fueling momentum.

- **Accountability**
  Get a friend or family member to check in on your progress. It's harder to skip a study session if you have to explain yourself. Online study groups or GRE forums can serve the same purpose.
- **Reward System**

  After a successful block of study (maybe four days in a row, no missed sessions), treat yourself. A dinner out, a new book—whatever gives you a little motivational spark.

3. Testing Yourself: The Benchmark Approach

There is no vantage point quite like the bird's-eye view you get from taking a full-length practice test. It forces you to juggle pacing, question variety, mental energy, and stress. If you're thinking you can waltz into the official GRE without doing *multiple* full simulations, brace for a harsh reality check.

- **Why Full Simulation Matters**

Consider endurance athletes: they train for race conditions because short sprints around the block don't replicate a true marathon. The GRE can last around four hours from check-in to final question. If your brain has never performed for that length, you might fade by the final verbal or quant section.

- **Data-Driven Adjustments**

Practice tests highlight your performance metrics. Are you consistently missing reading comprehension questions? Is your pacing too slow in the first 10 math questions, forcing you to guess on the last 5? Once you see the data, you can *fix* the problem.

- **Confidence Gains**

Confidence is not intangible. It's built from real, proven success in a timed environment. After you consistently score at or above your target in practice, you'll walk into test day with unstoppable self-belief.

4. Advanced Strategy and Mindset Tactics

A. The Art of Strategic Skipping

Sometimes the best way to *gain* points is by letting go of a few. If you see a question that's labyrinthine or heavy on advanced math you *barely* studied, consider skipping it momentarily. Reinvest that time in more straightforward questions. Then, circle back if time remains. It's better to ensure you grab certain points from simpler items than to risk them all on a single, time-sucking puzzle.

B. Focus on the Present Question

The GRE loves to create second-guessing. Maybe you bombed the last question—your mind is reeling. Or you got stuck halfway and had to guess. *Leave it behind.* Each new question is a fresh start. Let regrets go and give your full attention to the next item on your screen.

C. Use Whiteboard or Scratch Paper Wisely

For the GRE, you may have a certain type of scratch paper or an on-screen scratch pad. Don't scribble randomly. Keep track of question numbers if you do intermediate steps. This helps you check your work quickly if you have time at the end.

D. Gut Check for Tricky Questions

If you see a question with an immediate "trap answer" that looks too easy or lines up a bit *too* well with a "common misconception," pause. The test-makers know the typical mistakes. Usually, the real solution is more nuanced. Let your practiced instincts from your endless drills sniff out any suspicious freebies.

5. Addressing Test Anxiety

Even the calmest individuals can find the GRE stressful. After all, it's a high-stakes exam that influences your graduate school future. Use these proven anxiety-busters:

1. **Controlled Breathing**

If panic sets in, close your eyes (if permitted), inhale for four seconds, hold for four, and exhale for four. This slows your heart rate and clears your head.

2. **Positive Self-Talk**

This isn't fluffy self-help. Studies show that telling yourself "I've practiced this; I can do it" or "One question at a time" breaks destructive rumination patterns.

3. **Pre-Test Visualization**

Before you even enter the exam room, visualize yourself methodically tackling each question type. Your mind forms a mental script that can reduce the jolt of test-day nerves.

4. **Physical Prep**

Make sure you stay hydrated and not overly caffeinated. Caffeine can spike anxiety if you're already nervous. Balanced, stable energy is your friend.

6. The Final 24 Hours

When the clock is literally a day away from test day, it's time for a measured approach. Don't suddenly attempt 10 hours of cramming. Instead:

- **Light Review**

Quickly skim your key math formulas, your bullet-pointed notes on vocab, or your short list of grammar reminders.

- **No Intense Drills**

Full-length practice tests or complex problem sets might disrupt your mental balance. Trust that your prior training is enough.

- **Plan Your Logistics**

Double-check your route to the test center, your ID forms, watch, layers of clothes, healthy snacks, and water.

- **Early Bedtime**

Resist the temptation to burn the midnight oil. Freshness is more valuable than an extra hour of forced study.

This final day is about *confidence* and *calm.* Let your brain consolidate everything you've learned.

7. GRE Day Strategy

- **Arrive Early**
  You don't want to sprint through the door last minute. That spikes stress.
- **Check In**
  Have your IDs ready. Listen to the administrators' instructions.
- **Calm Start**

While waiting, do a final mental review of your pacing strategy: "I'll watch the clock every 5 questions. If I'm behind by a minute, I'll pick up the pace for the next 4 questions."

- **During the Test**
  - *Sections:* Attack each section with the fresh momentum it deserves.
  - *Breaks:* Use any official break to reset. Stretch, sip water. Avoid letting your mind swirl with self-doubt over the previous section.

When you finish, congratulate yourself. Win or lose, you gave it your best under a professional strategy. But given the preparation you've put in, expect a strong showing.

8. Mastering the Aftermath

Don't just vanish when the test is done. If you're not satisfied with your performance, dissect the experience:

- **What Surprised You?**

Maybe you realized you struggle with reading passages under time pressure more than in your practice. That's a sign your practice environment might need adjusting—fewer distractions, strict timers.

- **Were You Mentally Prepared?**

Did you get tired halfway through? Did you skip lunch? Did you properly handle your anxiety?

- **Retake Strategy**

If you must retake, design an even sharper plan. You'll now have direct, personal insight into the exam's demands.

9. Essential Tools: Revisited

Let's recap the most powerful items in your arsenal:

1. **Time-Awareness** – You always know how much time is left relative to how many questions remain.
2. **Strategic Guessing** – The $5 principle ensures that your random guesses remain random, while avoiding reckless eliminations.
3. **General Strategies** – Read carefully, benchmark answer choices, look out for pivot words.
4. **Top 20 Test Tips** – They are your final cheat sheet. Memorize them. Live by them.
5. **Focus and Calm** – You have no time for meltdown or second-guessing. One question at a time.

10. Parting Thoughts: Own Your Journey

By now, you recognize how multi-layered GRE success is. It's a puzzle requiring content knowledge, mental stamina, stealth time-management, and calm under pressure. But here's the good news: *None* of these elements are innate gifts. They are all *trainable* skills. Every single test-taker who invests the right amount of focus, practice, and reflection can dramatically improve their score.

The Real Secret?

You, the test-taker, are the secret weapon. Not a fancy formula, not a "magical" practice test. Your effort, your methodical approach, your discipline—these will pay off. The GRE wants you to believe it's unstoppable. Prove the test wrong by showing up bulletproof, with every angle covered.

Use these strategies. Embrace the guesswork approach that keeps you afloat when you face perplexing questions. Log your practice sessions. Celebrate small victories. Harness that momentum. By test day, you'll be a *machine*, unstoppable and confident.

Let the real GRE be your final victory lap.

You have all the knowledge and strategy to carve out the scores you need. So stop doubting, start trusting your method. This exam is big, but you are bigger. Let's do this.

GRE QUESTIONS

1. In his initial works, the playwright made physical disease **(i)** _________ factor in the action; from this, his early critics inferred that he had a predilection for focusing on **(ii)** _________ subject matter.

Blank (i)

A) a pivotal
B) a nonexistent
C) an obscure

Blank (ii)

D) recondite
E) uncomplicated
F) morbid

2. In searching for norms in the sense of authoritative standards of what **ought** to be, rather than in the sense of what is average and thus "normal," normative ethics aims to _________.

A) predict
B) mitigate
C) question
D) dictate
E) personalize

3. The reason minimum temperatures are going up more rapidly than maximums may involve cloud cover and evaporative cooling. Clouds tend to keep days cooler by reflecting sunlight, and nights warmer by **(i)** _________ loss of heat from Earth's surface. Greater amounts of moisture in the soil from additional precipitation and cloudiness **(ii)** _________ the daytime temperature increases because part of the solar energy is **(iii)** _________ the evaporation of that moisture.

Blank (i)

A) inhibiting
B) exacerbating
C) replicating

Blank (ii)

D) augment
E) mask
F) restrain

Blank (iii)

G) intensified by
H) unrelated to
I) used up in

4. The company's efforts to improve safety were apparently **(i)** _________, at least according to the company's own data, which showed that the **(ii)** _________ incidents with the potential to cause a serious accident declined significantly. Nevertheless, independent analysts argue that those statistics are **(iii)** _________. These analysts maintain that the company has consistently underestimated both the probability and the likely effects of accidents in the sensitive and poorly understood environment in which the company is operating.

Blank (i)

A) innovative
B) successful
C) frustrated

Blank (ii)

D) frequency of
E) impediments to
F) attention to

Blank (iii)

G) deceptive
H) testable
I) consistent

5. For most of the first half of the nineteenth century, science at the university was in _________ state, despite the presence of numerous luminaries.

A) a scintillating
B) a pathetic
C) a controversial
D) an incendiary
E) a veracious

6. The sight of a single actor portraying several characters in the same scene is no longer a shock to the average moviegoer, such special-effects trickery having become so _________.

A) expensive
B) specialized
C) sinister
D) commonplace
E) unreliable

7. The gaps in existing accounts of the playwright's life are not **(i)** _________, since much of the documentary evidence on which historians have relied is **(ii)** _________.

Blank (i)

A) trifling
B) obvious
C) implicit

Blank (ii)

D) credible
E) extant
F) incomplete

8. Researchers trying to make it possible to trace counterfeit documents to the printer that produced them are **(i)** _________ the fact that the rotating drums and mirrors inside laser printers are imperfect devices that leave unique patterns of banding in their output. Although these patterns are **(ii)** _________ to the naked eye, they can be **(iii)** _________ and analyzed by computer programs that the researchers have spent the past year devising.

Blank (i)

A) exploiting
B) facing
C) manipulating

Blank (ii)

D) invisible
E) obvious
F) unappealing

Blank (iii)

G) detected
H) implemented
I) generated

9. At their best, **(i)** _________ book reviews are written in defense of value and in the tacit hope that the author, having had his or her **(ii)** _________ pointed out, might secretly agree that the book could be improved.

Blank (i)

A) abstruse
B) adverse
C) hortatory

Blank (ii)

D) strengths
E) transgressions
F) assumptions

10. In a recent history of the Renaissance, by showing how the artistic efflorescence of that era was **(i)** _________ linked to its commercial vitality, Jardine demonstrated that the spirit of acquisitiveness may be **(ii)** _________ that of cultural creativity.

Blank (i)

A) questionably
B) intimately
C) skeptically

Blank (ii)

D) threatened by
E) inseparable from
F) comparable to

11. The figure-skating pair's convincing victory last week was particularly **(i)** _________ to their rivals, who were in peak form and complained privately about the judging. That the pair won when their rivals were **(ii)** _________ too is also impressive.

Blank (i)

A) unsurprising
B) irksome
C) gratifying

Blank (ii)

D) terrific
E) nervous
F) inconsistent

12. When she first came to France from Bulgaria, she was hardly the _________ student she later claimed to be, since she actually had access to substantial family wealth.

A) naïve
B) precocious
C) impecunious
D) ambitious
E) assiduous

13. Female labor was essential to the growth of eighteenth-century European textile industries, yet it remains difficult to **(i)** _________. Despite significant **(ii)** _________ in research about women, the role of female labor remains the single most glaring omission in most economic analyses of the history of European industrialization. Women far outnumbered men as workers in the textile industries, yet wage indices and discussions of growth, cost of living, and the like **(iii)** _________ about the male labor force.

Blank (i)

A) track
B) overestimate
C) ignore

Blank (ii)

D) advances
E) gaps
F) disinterest

Blank (iii)

G) incorporate data only
H) suppress most information
I) too rarely talk

14. The serious study of popular culture by intellectuals is regularly credited with having rendered obsolete a once-dominant view that popular culture is inherently inferior to high art. Yet this alteration of attitudes may be somewhat **(i)** _________. Although it is now academically respectable to analyze popular culture, the fact that many intellectuals feel compelled to rationalize their own **(ii)** _________ action movies or mass-market fiction reveals, perhaps unwittingly, their continued **(iii)** _________ the old hierarchy of high and low culture.

Blank (i)

A) counterproductive
B) underappreciated
C) overstated

Blank (ii)

D) penchant for
E) distaste for
F) indifference to

Blank (iii)

G) aversion to
H) investment in
I) misunderstanding of

15. In her startlingly original writing, she went further than any other twentieth-century author in English (perhaps in any language) in **(i)** _________ literary language and form, **(ii)** _________ stylistic conventions, and **(iii)** _________ a rich and diverse structure of meaning.

Blank (i)

A) reinventing
B) canonizing
C) stabilizing

Blank (ii)

D) undoing
E) overpraising
F) misunderstanding

Blank (iii)

G) replicating
H) borrowing
I) introducing

16. The setting in which the concert took place **(i)** _________: the group's performance was elegant and polished, but the sound, which seeped across the cold, unresonant high school auditorium, was oddly **(ii)** _________, given the energy the players seemed to be putting into it.

Blank (i)

A) exacted a toll
B) encouraged nervousness
C) solved a dilemma

Blank (ii)

D) clangorous
E) tepid
F) inviting

17. That today's students of American culture tend to **(i)** _________ classical music is understandable. In our own time, America's musical high culture has degenerated into a formulaic entertainment divorced from the contemporary moment. Thus, to miss out on what our orchestras are up to is not to **(ii)** _________ much. In the late Gilded Age, however, music was widely esteemed as the "queen of the arts." Classical music was in its American heyday, **(iii)** _________ the culture at large.

Blank (i)

A) promote
B) reinterpret
C) ignore

Blank (ii)

D) sacrifice
E) appreciate
F) malign

Blank (iii)

G) antagonistic toward
H) generally rejected by
I) centrally embedded in

18. For each of Questions 1 to 9, select one entry for each blank from the corresponding column of choices. Fill all blanks in the way that best completes the text.

This composer has never courted popularity: her rugged modernism seems to defy rather than to _________ the audience.

A) ignore
B) discount
C) woo
D) teach
E) cow

19. It is a sad but just indictment of some high school history textbooks that they frequently report as **(i)** _________ claims that historians hotly debate or that are even completely **(ii)** _________ by **(iii)** _________ primary sources.

Blank (i)

A) factual
B) controversial
C) sensational

Blank (ii)

D) resolved
E) corroborated
F) contradicted

Blank (iii)

G) dubious
H) incomplete
I) reliable

20. We have yet to **(i)** _________ the assessment of Canada's biodiversity. Most of the vertebrates have been assessed, but our challenge will be the assessment of invertebrates and plants. This task is **(ii)** _________ not only because of the high number of species, but also because of the diversity, each species requiring a different approach.

Blank (i) A) initiate
B) complete
C) limit

Blank (ii) D) repetitious
E) trivial
F) daunting

21. Researchers have observed chimpanzees feigning injury in order to influence other members of the group, thus showing that the capacity to _________ is not uniquely human.

A) cooperate
B) instruct

C) conspire
D) dissemble
E) dominate

22. Early studies often concluded that the public was _________ the propagandistic influence of mass communications, but one recent study indicates that, on the contrary, mass communications seldom produce marked changes in social attitudes or actions.

A) unaware of
B) scornful of
C) susceptible to
D) unimpressed by
E) coping with

23. The media once portrayed the governor as anything but ineffective; they now, however, make her out to be the epitome of _________.

A) fecklessness
B) brilliance
C) dynamism
D) egoism
E) punctiliousness

24. Instant celebrity is often **(i)** _________ asset because if there is no **(ii)** _________ to interest the public—no stage or screen triumphs, no interesting books, no heroic exploits—people quickly become bored.

Blank (i)

A) a fleeting
B) an incomparable
C) an untapped

Blank (ii)

D) competing attraction
E) continuity of exposure
F) real achievement

25. The governor has long been obsessed with excising the media from the relationship between politicians and the public. That has been the unifying purpose behind her otherwise seemingly unconnected efforts since taking office: a determination to **(i)** _________, and eventually **(ii)** _________, the media's hold on political communication.

Blank (i)

A) conceal
B) erode
C) rejuvenate

Blank (ii)

D) augment
E) consolidate
F) end

26. It was her view that the country's problems had been _______ by foreign technocrats, so that to ask for such assistance again would be counterproductive.

A. ameliorated
B. ascertained
C. diagnosed
D. exacerbated
E. overlooked
F. worsened

27. Reading Passage

"Reviving the practice of using elements of popular music in classical composition, an approach that had been in hibernation in the United States during the 1960s, composer Philip Glass (born 1937) embraced the ethos of popular music in his compositions. Glass based two symphonies on music by rock musicians David Bowie and Brian Eno, but the symphonies' sound is distinctively his. Popular elements do not appear out of place in Glass's classical music, which from its early days has shared certain harmonies and rhythms with rock music. Yet this use of popular elements has not made Glass a composer of popular music. His music is not a version of popular music packaged to attract classical listeners; it is high art for listeners steeped in rock rather than the classics."

Based on this passage, which quality does Glass's work exhibit?

A. A return to the use of popular music in classical compositions
B. An attempt to elevate rock music to an artistic status more closely approximating that of classical music
C. A long-standing tendency to incorporate elements from two apparently disparate musical styles

28. Text Completion

It is refreshing to read a book about our planet by an author who does not allow facts to be (i)__________ by politics: well aware of the political disputes about the effects of human activities on climate and biodiversity, this author does not permit them to (ii)__________ his comprehensive description of what we know about our biosphere. He emphasizes the enormous gaps in our knowledge, the sparseness of our observations, and the (iii)__________, calling attention to the many aspects of planetary evolution that must be better understood before we can accurately diagnose the condition of our planet.

For the blanks, choose from the following options:

Blank (i): A. overshadowed, B. invalidated, C. illuminated
Blank (ii): D. enhance, E. obscure, F. underscore
Blank (iii): G. plausibility of our hypotheses, H. certainty of our entitlement, I. superficiality of our theories

29. Although it does contain some pioneering ideas, one would hardly characterize the work as __________.

A. orthodox
B. eccentric
C. original
D. trifling
E. conventional
F. innovative

30. In parts of the Arctic, the land grades into the landfast ice so _______ that you can walk off the coast and not know you are over the hidden sea.

A. permanently
B. imperceptibly
C. irregularly

D. precariously
E. relentlessly

31. Reading Passage

"Reviving the practice of using elements of popular music in classical composition, an approach that had been in hibernation in the United States during the 1960s, composer Philip Glass (born 1937) embraced the ethos of popular music in his compositions. Glass based two symphonies on music by rock musicians David Bowie and Brian Eno, but the symphonies' sound is distinctively his. Popular elements do not appear out of place in Glass's classical music, which from its early days has shared certain harmonies and rhythms with rock music. Yet this use of popular elements has not made Glass a composer of popular music. His music is not a version of popular music packaged to attract classical listeners; it is high art for listeners steeped in rock rather than the classics."

Which issue regarding Glass's incorporation of popular elements in his classical pieces is discussed in the passage?

A. How it is regarded by listeners who prefer rock to the classics
B. How it has affected the commercial success of Glass's music
C. Whether it has contributed to a revival of interest among other composers in using popular elements in their compositions
D. Whether it has had a detrimental effect on Glass's reputation as a composer of classical music
E. Whether it has caused certain of Glass's works to be derivative in quality

32. Vain and prone to violence, Caravaggio could not handle success: the more his (i)__________ as an artist increased, the more (ii)__________ his life became.

For the blanks, choose from the following options:

Blank (i): A. temperance, B. notoriety, C. eminence
Blank (ii): D. tumultuous, E. providential, F. dispassionate

33. A school nurse measures the height of every boy in a school with 1000 pupils and determines that the average height is 1.64 meters with a standard deviation of 0.05 meter. Which of the following statements is true?

a. Sixty-eight percent of the students have heights between 1.59 meters and 1.69 meters.
b. There are as many students with heights above 1.64 meters as below 1.64 meters.

c. More students are 1.64 meters tall than any other height.
d. None of these statements may be made conclusively.

34. Suppose your actual weight is 150 pounds and you weigh yourself with an analog scale and get a reading of 152.1 pounds. You repeat the measurement twice more and get 152.1 pounds each time. Which of the following statements is true?

a. There is no random error.
b. There is no systematic error.
c. The systematic error is 2.1 pounds.
d. The random error is 2.1 pounds.

35. Which of the following numbers has the most significant digits?

a. 1,500,000
b. 1.5000 × 105
c. 0.15000
d. 0.00150000

36. An inch is approximately equivalent to which of the following?

a. 254 mm
b. 25.4 cm
c. 2.54 x 10-4 km
d. 2.54 x 102 m

37. Cobalt-63 can be produced in a laboratory and is unstable. When it decays, a neutron in its core will likely decay into a proton, changing Cobalt-63 into Nickel-63. Which of the following products will be produced when a neutron decays into a proton?

I. alpha particles
II. beta particle
III. gamma particles
a. I only
b. III only
c. II and III
d. I, II and III

38. What happens to a nucleus when it emits an alpha particle?

a. Its atomic number decreases by one.
b. Its mass decreases by two atomic mass units.
c. Its nucleon number decreases by four.
d. Its charge increases by +2.

39. Which of the following statements about isotopes of an element is true?

a. They have the same number of nucleons.
b. They have the same number of neutrons, but different numbers of protons.
c. They have the same number of protons, but different numbers of neutrons.
d. They have a different number of electrons.

40. How is energy generated in a nuclear reaction?

a. Matter is converted into energy.
b. Photon excitation and emission.
c. Kinetic collision of highly energetic hydrogen atoms.
d. Gravitational energy is converted into electromagnetic radiation.

41. How is light created in the core of the sun?

a. convection
b. fission reactions
c. fusion reactions
d. chemical reactions

42. A nucleus absorbs a neutron and undergoes a fission reaction. Which of the following statements explains why this happens?

a. The nucleus is more stable with the additional neutron.
b. The new nucleus is unstable.
c. Energy is released.
d. The binding energy per nucleon decreases.

43. A substance has a half-life of 2.4 × 104 years. How long does it take for 87.5% of the substance to decay?

a. 2.1 × 104 years
b. 4.5 × 104 years

c. 7.2 × 104 years
d. 9.6 × 104 years

44. A hydrogen atom makes a transition from the first excited state to the ground level. Which of the following statements is true?

a. A 10.2 eV photon is emitted.
b. A 13.6 eV photon is emitted.
c. A 1.9 eV photon is absorbed.
d. No photon is emitted.

45. What is the magnification of a combination of three lenses with magnifications 3.0, −4.0, and 0.3?

a. − 0.7
b. 0.7
c. − 3.6
d. 3.6

46. Which of the following statements is not a principle used in constructing ray diagrams to show the creation of images using a thin convex lens?

a. A ray parallel to the optical axis is refracted so that it goes through the focal point of the lens.
b. A ray that goes through the focal point of a lens and strikes the lens is refracted parallel to the optical axis.
c. A ray that goes through the center of a lens is not deflected.
d. A ray that strikes the surface of a lens follows Snell's law for refraction.

47. Which type of aberration does not occur with concave spherical mirrors?

a. Astigmatism
b. Chromatic aberration
c. Spherical aberration
d. Distortion

48. A thin convex lens has focal length of 30 cm. An identical lens is placed right behind it. What is the focal length of this combination of lenses?

a. 30 cm.
b. 60 cm

c. 15 cm
d. 0.067 cm

49. A lens forms an upright image 19 cm from a lens of an object 49 cm from the lens. The object and image are on the same side of the lens. What is the magnification of the image?

a. 0.39
b. 2.6
c. 13.7
d. 31.2

50. An object is 20 cm centimeters in front of a thin convex lens with a focal point of 10 centimeters. Where is the image located?

a. 10 cm in front of the lens.
b. 20 cm in front of the lens.
c. 10 cm behind the lens.
d. 20 cm behind the lens.

51. Which of the following statements about the image created by a magnifying glass is true?

a. The image is always upside down.
b. The image is always right side up.
c. The image may be right side up or upside down, depending on the location of the object.
d. The image may be right side up or upside down, depending on the thickness of the lens.

52. An object is placed a certain distance away from a convex spherical mirror. Which of the following statements is true?

a. No image is formed.
b. The image will be larger or smaller, depending on the object's distance from the mirror.
c. The image will be smaller and right side up.
d. The image will be smaller and either right side up or upside down, depending on the object's distance from the mirror.

53. Two rays parallel to the optical axis of a concave mirror are incident upon the mirror. Where do the two rays intersect?

a. At a point behind the mirror.
b. At infinity.

c. At the center of curvature.
d. At the focal point.

54. Which of the following theories best explains the phenomenon of total internal reflection?

a. The speed of light is a maximum in a vacuum.
b. Light consists of bundles of energy called photons.
c. Snell's law places a limit on the angle of refraction.
d. Light consists of transverse waves.

55. Which of the following statements explains what causes a rainbow?

a. The components of sunlight strike water droplets at different angles.
b. Water moles produce an emission spectrum when sunlight strikes them.
c. The speed of light in water depends on its wavelength.
d. There is total internal reflection for certain wavelengths of sunlight.

56. A ray of light travelling in a vacuum (n = 1) is incident upon a glass plate (n = 1.3). It hits with an angle of incidence of 45°. If the angle of incidence increases to 50°, what is the new angle of refraction?

a. It is 45°
b. It is 50°
c. It is below 45°
d. It is above 50°

57. Specular reflection might come occur on a surface like a mirror, while diffuse reflection might occur on a wooden tabletop. Which of the following statements best describes the difference between specular and diffuse reflection?

a. For diffuse reflection, the angle of incidence is equal to the angle of reflection.
b. For diffuse reflection, surface irregularities are large compared to the wavelength of visible light.
c. One hundred percent of the light is reflected for specular reflection.
d. The conservation of momentum is followed in specular reflection.

58. Which of the following phenomena is most closely related to the phenomenon that produces the light from lasers?

a. radioactivity
b. phosphorescence
c. sunlight
d. blackbody radiation

59. Which of the following phenomena implies that light consists of specific quanta?

a. ultraviolet catastrophe
b. threshold frequency
c. emission of light
d. stability of atoms

60. Which of the following statements best explains why light is polarized?

a. Light waves' electromagnetic fields can be oriented in a particular direction by a polarizer.
b. Photons of light can be pointed in the same direction by microscopic holes in a polarizer.
c. Light travels in a vacuum.
d. Light is a longitudinal wave.

61. Which of the following is true about a diffraction grating?

a. The more slits per inch, the greater the amount of destructive interference.
b. Blue light diffracts more than red light in a diffraction grating.
c. A diffraction grating produces maxima and minima only for monochromatic light.
d. Light passing through a diffraction grating produces a bulls-eye pattern.

62. When light from a single source strikes two slits, alternating bright and dark lines appear on a screen on the far side. What is the best explanation for this phenomenon?

a. Doppler shift
b. Diffraction and interference
c. Chromatic aberration
d. Total internal reflection

63. Two beams of light with the same phase and wavelength travel different paths and arrive at the same point. If maximum constructive interference occurs at this point, which of the following statements is true?

a. The two beams arrive 180° out of phase.
b. The two beans arrive 90° out of phase.

c. The lengths of the paths differ by an odd-number of half wavelengths.

d. The lengths of the paths differ by an integral number of wavelengths.

64. A homemade generator rotates at a constant frequency and produces an alternating current with a maximum voltage of 40 volts. It is connected to a resistor of 20 ohms. What is the average current that flows through the resistor?

a. 0 amperes.

b. 1.4 amperes

c. 2.0 amperes

d. 2.8 amperes

65. A miniature heater has a power rating of 50 watts and is connected to a battery with an electromotive force of 10 volts. What current flows through the heater?

a. 500 amperes

b. 5 amperes

c. 200 milliamperes

d. 3.1 × 1019 electrons per second

66. A 6.0-megaohm resistor is connected in series with a 5.0-microfarad capacitor and fully charged with a 3-volt battery. The battery is disconnected and the capacitor is connected directly to the resistor. How long will it take for the capacitor to fully discharge?

a. Infinite time

b. 30 seconds

c. 0.0333 second

d. 90 seconds

67. A 5-microfarad and a 15-microfarad capacitor are connected as shown in the diagram. What is the total capacitance of the circuit?

5 μF

|

|

15 μF

a. 3.8 μF

b. 3 μF

c. 20 μF

d. 75 μF

68. Adding multiple capacitors to a circuit is much the opposite as adding multiple resistors. Adding resistors in series, for example, creates an effective resistance equal to their sum. To add resistors in parallel, you must add the reciprocals of their resistance. With capacitors, however, you use reciprocals when adding them in series and you sum the capacitance when adding in parallel. Given the following diagram, what is the total capacitance of the circuit?

3 μF 6 μF

a. 2-microfarads

b. 9-microfarads

c. 0.5-microfarads

d. 4.5 microfarads

69. Which is the correct formula for the energy stored in a fully-charged capacitor with capacitance C when its attached to a battery of voltage V?

a. C/V

b. ½CV2

c. CV

d. 0 volt

70. A capacitor is connected in series to a battery and a resistor. The battery is disconnected after the capacitor is charged and replaced by a battery with a greater electromotive force, causing the capacitor to gain additional charge. After the capacitor has fully charged again, which of the following statements is true about the capacitance of the circuit?

a. It has increased.

b. It has decreased.

c. It has remained the same.

d. It has become zero.

71. Consider one tungsten wire of length L and cross-sectional area A and another tungsten wire of length 2L and area 2A. Assuming both wires are the same temperature, which of the following statements is true?

a. The resistance of the two wires is the same.

b. The resistance of the longer wire is twice the resistance of the shorter wire.

c. The resistance of the longer wire is half the resistance of the shorter wire.
d. The resistance of the longer wire is four times the resistance of the shorter wire.

72. What is the total resistance between points X and Y in the circuit diagram below?

```
            X
            |
          10-Ω
            |
       |---- 3-Ω ----
       |            |
  |---- 2-Ω ----   4-Ω
            |
            Y
```

a. 0 Ω
b. 12 Ω
c. 19 Ω
d. 16 Ω

73. A circuit consists of a battery and a resistor. An ammeter is used to measure the current in the circuit and is connected in series to the circuit. Which of the following is true?

a. The current flowing in the resistor increases.
b. The current flowing in the resistor decreases.
c. The voltage drop across the resistor increases.
d. The current flowing in the resistor remains the same.

74. Which of the following statements about electricity flowing through a circuit can be correctly derived from Ohm's law?

a. Increasing the voltage decreases the current if the resistance remains unchanged.
b. Increasing the current and the resistance decreases the voltage.
c. Increasing the current increases the voltage if the resistance is unchanged.
d. Decreasing the resistance increases the current if the voltage remains unchanged.

75. Which of the following devices changes chemical energy into electrical energy?

a. battery
b. closed electric circuit

c. generator
d. transformer

76. Current in an electrical circuit is normally measured in amperes. Which of the following does not represent an alternative way of expressing units of current?

a. coulombs per second
b. volts per ohm
c. electrons per second
d. Watt-volts.

77. The diagram below shows two batteries connected in series to a resistor. What is the direction of current flow?

a. clockwise
b. counterclockwise
c. neither clockwise nor counterclockwise
d. Can't be determined from the information given.

78. Which of the following gives the correct order of electromagnetic radiation from the lowest frequency to the highest frequency?

a. microwaves, UHF radio waves, x-rays, visible light
b. UHF radio waves, microwaves, visible light, x-rays
c. UHF radio waves, microwaves, visible light, x-rays
d. microwaves, x-rays, visible light, UHF radio waves

79. Electromagnetic radiation — also known as light — consists of perpendicularly oscillating electric and magnetic fields. Which of the following statements about electromagnetic radiation is untrue?

a The energy of the radiation is determined by the frequency and Plank's constant.
b. The "color" of light is determined by its wavelength.
c. Electromagnetic radiation sometimes obeys wave theory.
d. Electromagnetic radiation sometimes obeys particle theory.

80. In the 19th century, James Clerk Maxwell calculated the speed of light in a vacuum from the proportionality constants used in electrostatics and magnetism. Which of the following relationships correctly identifies how light moves in a vacuum?

a. High frequencies of light travel faster than low frequencies.
b. Low frequencies of light travel faster than high frequencies.
c. All frequencies of light travel at the same speed in a vacuum.
d. Light moves at infinite speed through a vacuum.

81. A solenoid is made of loops of wire, through which a current is run. What is the purpose of putting a lot of loops into a solenoid?

a. To increase the magnetic field inside the solenoid.
b. To increate the magnetic field outside the solenoid.
c. To decrease the magnetic field inside the solenoid.
d. To decrease the magnetic field outside the solenoid.

82. An electron is moving in a straight line. Another particle is moving in a straight line parallel to the path of the electron but in the opposite direction. Initially the electron and particle are far apart, but get closer together. When the two particles are in the vicinity of one another, they experience an attractive magnetic force. Which of the following is a correct inference from this fact?

a. The particle has a north pole and a south pole.
b. The particle is positively charged.
c. The particle is negatively charged.
d. The particle has either a north pole or a south pole.

83. The charged particle moving through a magnetic field will be subject to a force of $F = qvB \operatorname{Sin}\theta$, where q is the charge, v is the particle's velocity, B is the magnetic field strength, and θ is the particle's angle between the magnetic field vector and the velocity vector. Charged particles from space enter the earth's atmosphere all the time. For example, the Aurora Borealis or Northern Lights are created by positive and negative charges passing through the Earth's magnetic field. Assume a proton with a speed of 8.0 × 106 meters per second enters the Earth's magnetic field at an angle of 45°, at a point where the magnetic field is 0.5 Teslas. What is the magnetic force acting on the proton? Note: the proton has a charge of 1.6 × 10−19 coulombs.

a. 6.4 × 10−17 newtons
b. 4.5 × 10−17 newtons
c. 4.5 × 10−13 newtons
d. 5.5 × 10−17 tesla

84. Which law says the number of electric field lines passing through an imaginary surface is proportional to the net charge inside the surface?

a. Coulomb's law
b. Gauss's law
c. Faraday's law of induction
d. Biot-Savart law

85. A plastic comb is used to comb someone's dry hair and acquires a large positive charge. The comb is brought close to a small bit of uncharged paper lying on a table. Against the force of gravity, the bit of paper jumps up and sticks to the comb. What is likely to happen next?

a. The paper will stick to the comb indefinitely.
b. Air will eventually cause the comb to lose its charge and the paper will fall from the comb under the force of gravity.
c. The paper will acquire a positive charge and be repelled by the comb.
d. The paper will acquire a negative charge and be repelled by the comb.

86. When is the potential of a point charge with respect to a dipole equal to 0 volts per coulomb?

a. At the midpoint between the positive and negative charge.
b. At an infinite distance from the dipole.
c. At the negative charge.
d. At the positive charge.

87. An electric field is pointing from south to north. If a dipole is placed in the field, how will the dipole's orientation change?

a. The positive charge will be on the northern side and the negative charge will be on the southern side.
b. The positive charge will be on the southern side and the negative charge will be on the northern side.
c. The positive charge will be on the eastern side and the negative charge will be on the western side.
d. There will be no change in the orientation.

88. Which of the following is true of an electric dipole?

a. They don't exist in nature.
b. The charges are equal in magnitude and both are negative.

c. The charges have opposite signs and can be unequal in magnitude.
d. The charges are equal in magnitude and have opposite signs.

89. An electron moves in a uniform electric field in the same direction as the electric field from point A to point B. Which of the following statements is true?

a. The potential energy of the electron decreased
b. The potential energy of the electron
c. The potential energy of the electron remained constant
d. The potential energy of the electron was converted into kinetic energy

90. Which of the following statements about a solid metal sphere with a net charge is true?

a. If the charge is positive, it will be distributed uniformly throughout the sphere.
b. The charge will be distributed uniformly at the surface of the sphere.
c. The charge will leave the sphere.
d. The electric field will be tangent to the surface of the sphere.

91. Which of the following statements best describes the electric field shown below.

a. The field is decreasing down.
b. The field is decreasing to the right.
c. The field is increasing to the right.
d. The field is uniform.

92. A charge +2q is placed at the origin of a coordinate system and a charge of -q is placed at a distance d from the origin. How far from the origin must a third charge +q be placed so that the net force on it is 0 newtons?

a. Less than d/2
b. Between d/2 and d
c. Between d and 2d
d. Greater than 2d

93. Which of the following is the correct definition of a conductor?

a. A metal wire in an electrical circuit.
b. A material that contains movable electric charges.
c. A material that is not a semiconductor or insulator.
d. Any device that allows electricity to flow.

94. What does it mean when someone says that electric charge is conserved?

a. Like charges repel, and unlike charges attract.
b. The net charge of an isolated system remains constant.
c. Charges come from electrons and protons.
d. Charge can never be created or destroyed.

95. An object with a net charge is brought into the vicinity of an object with a net charge of zero coulombs. Which statement describes the electrostatic force between the two objects?

a. It is a repulsive force.
b. It is an attractive force.
c. There is no force.
d. It is a perpendicular force.

96. A cube of a substance is 5 centimeters on each side. It is placed in a pressure chamber where the pressure on each surface is 3.0 × 107 N/m2, causing the density of the cube increases by 0.01 %. Which of the following theories is used to describe this?

a. Young's Modulus
b. Shear Modulus
c. Elastic modulus
d. Bulk Modulus

97. Which statement best explains why water expands when it freezes?

a. The coefficient of thermal expansion is negative.
b. The average distance between the water molecules increases.
c. The density of water is greater at higher temperatures.
d. The internal energy of the water decreases.

98. Which statement correctly describes the elastic limit of a metal rod?

a. The elastic limit occurs when a deformed object will no longer return to its original shape.
b. The elastic limit occurs when the rod breaks.
c. The elastic limit occurs when the stress stops producing a strain.
d. The elastic limit assumes that the forces between molecules in a metal act like springs.

99. A cube of aluminum is placed at the bottom of a deep ocean where the pressure is over 20 atmospheres. What happens to the density of the cube?

a. It remains the same.
b. It decreases slightly.
c. It increases slightly.
d. It becomes zero.

100. The air passing over an airplane's wind is considered an irrotational fluid flow. Which of the following statements correctly describes the concept of irrotational fluid flow?

a. The fluid flows in a straight line.
b. All particles have the same velocity as they pass a particular point.
c. A tiny paddle wheel placed in the fluid will rotate.
d. The fluid does not have any rotating points, whirlpools or eddies.

101. An incompressible ideal fluid flows through a pipe 5.0 cm in radius at a speed of 6.0 m/s. The pipe narrows to 3.0 cm. What is the speed of flow in the narrower section?

a. 10 m/s
b. 3.6 m/s
c. 16.7 m/s
d. Can't be determined from the given information.

102. Suppose you have a pipe of length L and radius r, and a liquid with viscosity η. You also have a sensor to detect the liquid's flow rate, which measures the volume of liquid passing through the pipe per second. If you want to increase the pipe's flow rate, what changes to L, r and η should you make? Assume that the pressure differential remains constant.

a. Increase L, increase r, and decreases η
b. Decrease L, increase r, and decreases η
c. Decrease L, increase r, and increase η
d. Increase L, decrease r, and decreases η

103. The center of a circular aquarium window with a radius 1 meter is 14 meters below the surface. What is the force of the water at this depth pushing on this window? The density of water is 1000 kg/m3.

a. 1.37 × 105 newtons
b. 1.08× 105 newtons

c. 4.3 × 105 newtons

d. 0 newtons

104. A hydraulic lift needs to raise a 3.5 × 103 newton truck. The input piston has a diameter of 2.0 cm and the output piston has a diameter of 24 cm. What minimum force must be applied to the input piston?

a. 24 N

b. 292 N

c. 42,000 N

d. 504,000 N

105. A submarine sits underwater at a constant depth of 50 meters. Which of the following is true about the submarine's buoyant force?

a. It is 0 N.

b. It is greater than 0 N but less than the submarine's weight

c. It is equal to the submarine's weight

d. It is greater than the submarine's weight

106. Substance A has a density of 5.0 kg/m3 and substance B has a density of 4.0 kg/m3. What is the ratio of the volume A to volume B when the masses of the two substances are equal?

a. 1.25

b. 0.80

c. 1.12

d. 0.89

107. Ultrasound imaging, which is used for various medical procedures, including imaging pregnant women, is based on which of the following principles.

a. Doppler effect.

b. Echolocation

c. Infrasonic.

d. Resonance.

108. The speed of a travelling wave in a stretched string is given by $\sqrt{(T/\mu)}$, where T is the tension in the string and μ is the mass per unit length. A 2-meter-long stretched string with a mass of 0.010 kilograms is made to resonate with standing waves at 50 Hz. What tension in the string is needed to produce the fourth harmonic? (Note: the fourth harmonic fits 2 full waves into the length of the string).

a. 12. 5 newtons
b. 25 newtons
c. 50 newtons
d. 10,000 newtons

109. In musical instruments with two open ends, the first harmonic fits one-half wave inside the tube. The second harmonic fits 1 full wave in the tube. The third harmonic fits 1.5 full waves in the tube. Etc. An organ pipe, open at both ends, has a length of 1.2 meters. What is the frequency of the third harmonic? The speed of sound is 340 meters per second.

a. 142 Hz
b. 284 Hz
c. 425 Hz
d. 568 Hz

110. What property of a sound wave in air corresponds to the frequency of the sound?

a. pitch
b. high and low
c. timbre
d. overtones

111. The density of helium is much lower than that of air. How does the speed of sound traveling through helium gas compare to the speed of sound in air?

a. It is faster
b. It is slower
c. It is the same speed
d. It cannot be determined without knowing their atomic masses

112. What corresponds to the amplitude of a sound wave?

a. loudness
b. pressure differential of fluctuations
c. magnitude of motion of air molecules
d. power

113. Which of the following statements about refraction is true.

a. Refraction means a change in direction of the wave.
b. The angle of reflection equals the angle of refraction.
c. The frequency in a refracted wave changes.
d. The phase of a refracted wave changes.

114. Two tuning forks have a frequency of 500 Hz and 504 Hz and the same amplitude. How much time is there between beats?

a. 4 seconds
b. 15 seconds
c. 0.25 seconds
d. 2 seconds

115. Transverse travelling waves propagate through a taut string of length 20 meters at a speed of 4 m/s. Standing waves are set up in this string which is fixed at both ends. What is the smallest frequency possible for the standing waves?

a. 0.1 Hz
b. 0.05 Hz
c. 0.2 Hz
d. 0.4 Hz

116. In resonance, small vibrations can produce a larger standing wave that becomes stronger than the original vibrations, assuming the vibrations are at the right frequency to generate resonance. If a pendulum is vibrated at a resonance frequency, what would you expect to happen?

a. The period of the pendulum will increase.
b. The time between swings will decrease.
c. The pendulum will swing higher.
d. The length of the pendulum will decrease.

117. Two waves, each of which has an amplitude of A, cross paths. At the point where they cross, the peak of one wave meets the trough of another wave. What is the resulting amplitude at the point where the waves cross?

a. 0
b. A

c. 2A

d. -A

118. What is the speed of a wave with a frequency of 12 Hz and a wavelength of 3 meters?

a. 12 meters per second

b. 36 meters per second

c. 4 meters per second

d. 0.25 meters per second

119. A RADAR gun sends out a pulsed beam of microwave radiation to measure the speed of cars using the Doppler effect. The pulsed beam bounces off the moving car and returns to the RADAR gun. For a car that's moving away from the RADAR detector, which of the following statements about the pulsed beam are true?

I. It returns with a longer wavelength.

II. It returns with a shorter wavelength.

III. It returns with a higher frequency.

a. I only.

b. II only.

c. I and III.

d. II and III.

120. Which of the following statements is true about the acceleration of a simple pendulum?

a. The acceleration is constant.

b. The magnitude of the acceleration is at a maximum when the bob is at the bottom of the path.

c. The magnitude of the acceleration is at a maximum when the bob is changing directions.

d. None of the above.

121. The equation for the amplitude of the motion of an object undergoing simple harmonic motion is A sin[(5.0 Hz)t]. Assuming the wave's phase is measured in radians, what is the period of the motion?

a. Sin [(5.0 Hz)t]

b. 2.5 seconds

c. 1.26 seconds

d. A

122. A 100-kg bungee jumper jumps off a bridge, attached to a 20 meter bungee cord. After bouncing around for a minute he finally comes to rest. The stretched cord is now 25 meters long. What is the spring constant of the bungee cord?

a. 20 newtons per meter
b. 39 newtons per meter
c. 49 newtons per meter
d. 196 newtons per meter

123. Which of the following statements best explains what is meant by the phase of a wave?

a. The height of a wave in 2π radians.
b. The length of a wave in 2π radians.
c. The period of oscillation of a wave.
d. An angle indicating the wave cycle's instantaneous location.

124. How much does it cost to operate a 5 kilowatt electric motor for 12 hours if electricity is 6 cents per kilowatt-hour?

a. $0.025
b. $3.60
c. $14.4
d. $360

125. Conservative forces are forces that do not lose energy to processes like friction and radiation and where the total mechanical energy is conserved. Which statement best explains why the work done by a conservative force on an object does not depend on the path the object takes?

a. This is the definition of a conservative force.
b. The work done by the force of friction on an object depends on the distance the object moves.
c. Work can be positive, negative, or zero.
d. If a force is conservative, any component of the force is equal to the change in a potential energy divided by the change in position.

126. Which of the following statements about energy is true?

a. Mechanical energy is always conserved in an isolated system.
b. Total energy is always conserved in an isolated system.

c. Energy is never created or destroyed.
d. You can determine the mechanical energy of an object by using E = mc2

127. Two objects of masses m and M are a distance R apart. The force of their gravitational attraction is given by GmM/R2. Their gravitational potential energy is given by -GmM/R. If the distance between these two objects doubles from 100 km to 200 km, what happens to the ratio of the gravitational force to the gravitational potential energy?

a. Doubled
b. Quadrupled
c. Halved
d. Quartered

128. The potential energy of a spring is represented as ½kx2, where k represents the spring constant and x is the displacement of the spring from its position when it is not stretched. A massless spring is suspended from a support and a 100-g mass is attached, stretching it 2 centimeters. If another 100-g mass is attached, what is the new potential energy of the spring?

a. Half as much as with one 100-g mass attached.
b. One-forth as much as with one 100-g mass attached.
c. Twice as much as with one 100-g mass attached.
d. Four times as much as with one 100-g mass attached.

129. A ball is released from a certain height along a frictionless track that does a loop-the-loop. The loop-the-loop part of the track is a perfect circle of radius R. At what height above the ground must the ball be released from in order to not fall off the track when it gets to the top of the loop-the-loop?

a. R
b. 2R
c. 2.5 R
d. 3R

130. A motorcycle weighs twice as much as a bicycle and is moving twice as fast. Which of the following statements is true?

a. The motor cycle has four times as much kinetic energy as the bicycle.
b. The motor cycle has eight times as much kinetic energy as the bicycle.

c. The bicycle and the motorcycle have the same kinetic energy.
d. The bicycle has four times as much kinetic energy as the motorcycle.

131. An athlete's foot is in contact with a kicked football for 100 milliseconds and exerts a force on the football over a distance of 20 centimeters. The force starts at 0 N and increases linearly to 2000 N for 50 milliseconds through a distance of 10 centimeters and then decreases linearly for 50 milliseconds through a distance of 10 centimeters. What is the average power of the athlete's foot while it is in contact with the ball?

a. 2 kilowatts
b. 4 kilowatts
c. 2000 kilowatts
d. 4000 kilowatts

132. Which statement correctly states the work-energy theorem?

a. The change in kinetic energy of an object is equal to the work done by the object.
b. The change in kinetic energy of an object is equal to the work done on an object.
c. The change in potential energy of an object is equal to the work done by the object.
d. The change in potential energy of an object is equal to the work done on an object.

133. Which statement best explains why the work done by a gravitational force on an object does not depend on the path the object takes.

a. Work depends on the path when there is friction. The longer the path the more energy is required to overcome friction.
b. Gravitational fields that arise from the interaction between point masses always produce elliptical paths of motion.
c. A falling object experiences a change in potential energy.
d. When an object falls down the work done by gravity is positive and when an object is thrown up the work done by gravity is negative.

134. A teacher pulls a box across the floor at a uniform speed. He pulls it with a spring scale showing that the force of kinetic friction is 2 newtons. How much total work is done in moving the box 5 meters?

a. 0 joules
b. 0.4 joules

c. 10 joules
d. 20 joules

135. A 75-kg ice skater moving eastward at 5 m/s collides with a 100-kg skater moving northward at 4 m/s. Anticipating the collision, they hug each other and produce an inelastic collision. What is their final speed?

a. Can't be determined from the information given.
b. 3.1 m/s
c. 4.1 m/s
d. 2.1 m/s

136. A bowling ball with a mass of 4 kilograms moving at a speed of 10 meters per second hits a stationary 1 kg bowling ball in a head-on elastic collision. What is the speed of the stationary ball after the collision?

a. 0 m/s
b. 10 m/s.
c. Less than 10 m/s, but not 0 m/s.
d. More than 10 m/s

137. Suppose a moving railroad car collides with an identical stationary car and the two cars latch together. Ignoring friction, and assuming no deformation on impact, which of the following statements is true?

a. The speed of the first car decreases by half.
b. The collision is elastic.
c. The speed of the first car is doubled.
d. There is no determining the final speed because the collision was inelastic.

138. Impulse is measured as the change in an object's momentum. Which statement is correct about the impulse on a ball rolling down a hill? Ignore air resistance and friction.

a. The impulse is constant.
b. The impulse only exists for a short time.
c. The units of impulse are joules per second.
d. The object's impulse increases.

139. Two cars driving in opposite directions collide. If you ignore friction and any other outside interactions, which of the following statements is always true?

a. The total momentum is conserved.
b. The sum of the potential and kinetic energy are conserved.
c. The total velocity of the cars is conserved.
d. The total impulse is conserved.

140. Astronauts in orbit are sometimes considered to be "weightless." Consider the four propositions about weightlessness and determine which ones are true.

I. Weightlessness occurs in outer space because the force of gravity becomes negligible.
II. Weightlessness occurs when a ski jumper makes a jump.
III. Weightlessness occurs when you roll a baseball on the ground.
a. I only.
b. II only.
c. I and II.
d. I, II and III.

141. Which has a greater moment of inertia about an axis through its center: a solid cylinder or a hollow cylinder? Both cylinders have the same mass and radius.

a. Solid cylinder
b. Hollow cylinder
c. Both have same moment of inertia.
d. It depends on how quickly the cylinders are rolling.

142. You blow up a rubber balloon and hold the opening tight with your fingers. You then release your fingers, causing air to blow out of the balloon. This pushes the balloon forward, causing the balloon shoots across the room. Which of Newton's laws best explains the cause of this motion?

a. First law
b. Second law
c. Third law
d. Law of gravity

143. Two unequal masses are balanced on a fulcrum using a massless bar, as shown below. If both masses are shifted towards the fulcrum so that their distances from the fulcrum are one-half the original distance, what happens to the masses?

a. The heavier mass will tilt downward.
b. The masses will remain balanced.
c. Cannot be determined from the information given.
d. The lighter mass will tilt downward.

144. A piece of art of mass 200 kg is suspended from two nails so that the angle the hanging wires make is 40° with the horizontal. What is the tension in the hanging wires? (Note: Sin 40° = 0.64 and Cos 40° = 0.77).

a. 1279 N
b. 1524 N
c. 1960 N
d. 3048 N

145. A force of 25.0 N pulls three blocks connected by a string on a frictionless surface. What is the tension in the rope between the 4.0-kg block and the 2.0-kg block? 4.0 kg — 2.0 kg — 3.0 kg

a. 0 N
b. 11.1 N
c. 16.7 N
d. 25 N

146. The pulley in the device below has no mass and is frictionless. The larger mass is 30 kg and the smaller mass is 20 kg. What is the acceleration of the masses?

a. 0.5 m/s2
b. 2 m/s2
c. 9.8 m/s2
d. 98 m/s2

147. The ideal mechanical advantage (IMA) of a pulley system indicates how much force is required to lift a mass. A fixed pulley has an IMA of 1 because all it only changes the direction of the force. A floating pulley has an IMA of 2. The total IMA is the product of the individual pulleys' IMAs. What is the ideal mechanical advantage of the pulley system below?

a. 1
b. 2
c. 3
d. 4

148. A 10-kg plastic block is at rest on a flat wooden surface. The coefficient of static friction between wood and plastic is 0.6 and the coefficient of kinetic friction is 0.5. How much horizontal force is needed to start the plastic box moving?

a. 5 N
b. 49 N
c. 59 N
d. 98 N

149. Bobsled tracks are flat when they are going straight, but when there is a turn, the track is angled (banked) to create a centripetal force. Assuming no friction, the banking angle is θ, the radius of curvature is r, and the maximum speed the bobsled can have without moving off the track is v. If the radius of curvature is doubled and the banking angle remains the same, which of the following statements is true?

a. The maximum speed is 2v.
b. The maximum speed is 4v.
c. The maximum speed is 1.4v.
d. The maximum speed depends on the banking angle.

150. In an amusement park ride, you stand on the floor of a cylindrical ring with your back touching the wall. The ring begins to rotate, slowly at first, but then faster and faster. When the ring is rotating fast enough, the floor is removed. You do not slide down but remained pressed against the wall of the ring. Which is the best explanation for why you don't fall down?

a. The centripetal force pushes you towards the wall.
b. The centripetal force changes the direction of your motion.
c. The force of friction between the wall and your body is greater than your weight.
d. The rotating ring creates a weightless environment.

151. A lead sphere 10 centimeters in diameter is attached to a 10-meter wire and suspended from a beam in a large warehouse. A lead sphere 1 meter in diameter is placed next to the smaller sphere, almost touching. Ignoring friction, which statement is true?

a. The small sphere will move slightly towards the big sphere, but the big sphere will not move.
b. The big sphere will move slightly toward the small sphere, but the small sphere will not move.
c. Neither sphere will move.
d. Both spheres will move slightly towards each other.

152. A box with a weight of 10 newtons is resting on a table. Which statement is true?

a. The force of the table on the box is the reaction to the weight of the box.
b. The force of the box on the table is the reaction to the weight of the box.
c. A 10 newton force on Earth is the reaction force.
d. There is no reaction force because the system is in equilibrium.

153. Consider the following statements about Newton's law:

I. A newton is a fundamental unit.
II. Mass and acceleration are inversely related when the force is constant.
III. Newton's first law can be derived from Newton's second law.
IV. Newton's second law can be derived from the universal law of gravity.
Which of the following statements are true?
a. I, II, and III.
b. II and III only.
c. III only.
d. I, II, III, and IV are not true.

154. Which of the following demonstrations best illustrates Newton's first law?

a. Giving a billiard ball at rest on a smooth level table a small push and letting it roll on the table.
b. Dragging a box on a table at a constant speed by exerting a force just enough to overcome the force of friction.
c. Trying without success to move a heavy bureau or filing cabinet on the floor.
d. Running a current through two parallel wires.

155. A space station is revolving in a circular orbit around Earth. Consider the following three statements:

I. The center of mass of the space station is necessarily located at its geometric center.
II. The center of mass is moving at a constant velocity.

III. The center of mass of the space station is moving at a constant speed.
Which of the following statements is true?

a. I is true.
b. II is true.
c. III is true.
d. I, II, and III are not true.

156. You throw a baseball straight up near the surface of Earth and it falls back to the ground. Which statement is true about the acceleration of the baseball at the top of its path? [Ignore air resistance]

a. The acceleration is zero.
b. The acceleration changes sign.
c. The acceleration is -9.8 m/s2.
d. The acceleration continues to increase.

157. An automobile increased its speed uniformly from 20 m/s to 30 m/s at rate 5 m/s2. During this time it traveled 50 meters. How long did it take the automobile to make this change?

a. 5 seconds
b. 2 seconds
c. 10 seconds
d. Can't be determined.

158. A perfectly circular track has a circumference of 400 meters. A runner goes around the track in 100 seconds instead of her usual time of 80 seconds because a leg cramp causes her to stop running for 20 seconds. What is her average speed?

a. 0 m/s
b. 5 m/s
c. 4 m/s
d. 20 m/s

159. A person walks 4 meters in a single direction. He or she then changes directions and walks an additional 9 meters. What is the total magnitude of the displacement of the person?

a. It is 13 meters.
b. It is always larger than 9 meters but less than 13 meters.

c. It is less than 13 meters and as small as 5 meters.
d. It is less than 5 meters.

160. Which of the following is a vector quantity?

a. Distance
b. Speed
c. Velocity
d. Time

161. The masses of four different objects taken with different scales were 23.04 g, 7.12 g, 0.0088 g and 5.423 g. What is the total mass of all four objects to the proper number of significant digits?

a. 35.59180
b. 35.5918
c. 35.60
d. 35.59

162. Which of the following measurements has the most significant digits?

a. 0.2990
b. 2.9900
c. 2.997
d. 0.00209

163. If $1<p<3$, then which of the following could be true?

I. $p2<2p$
II. $p2=2p$
III. $p2>2p$

(A) I only
(B) II only
(C) III only
(D) I and II only
(E) I, II, and III

164. Given the equation $x+2y=7$, which of the following could be the value of x?

(A) $x=0$
(B) $x=2$
(C) $x=3$
(D) $x=5$
(E) $x=7$

165. The product of which three of the following numbers is the greatest?

(A) -9
(B) -5
(C) -3
(D) 0
(E) 4
(F) 7
(G) 10

166. If *y, x,* and *z* are related in a figure, which of the following must be true?

(A) $y=z$
(B) $y<z$
(C) $y=x$
(D) $y>z$
(E) $y+z=2x$

167. If ABCD is a square, and OB is a radius of a circle. If BC is a tangent to the circle and PC = 2, what is the area of the square?

168. If ABCD is a rectangle, and F and E are points on AB and BC, respectively. The area of $\triangle DFB$ is 9 and the area of $\triangle BED$ is 24. What is the perimeter of the rectangle?

(A) 18
(B) 23
(C) 30
(D) 42
(E) 48

169. If ABCD is a square, and BCP is an equilateral triangle. What is the measure of *x*?

(A) 7.5
(B) 15

(C) 30
(D) 45
(E) 60

170. After a 20% discount, a calculator sells for $10. What was its original price?

(A) $20
(B) $12.5
(C) $12
(D) $9
(E) $7

171. Solve for *x* in the equation:

$$\frac{x+5}{x+1} = 4$$

(A) $\frac{1}{5}$
(B) $\frac{1}{2}$
(C) 1
(D) 5
(E) 10

172. In the system of equations:

$3x+4y=c$

$kx+12y=36$

If $k=9$ and $c=12$, and *x* and *y* are integers, which of the following could be *y*?
(A) -6
(B) 0
(C) 4
(D) 5
(E) 12

173. The ratio of chickens to pigs to horses on Richard's farm is 33:17:21. What fraction of the animals are either pigs or horses?

(A) $\frac{16}{53}$
(B) $\frac{17}{54}$
(C) $\frac{38}{71}$
(D) $\frac{25}{31}$
(E) $\frac{38}{33}$

174. The angles in $\triangle ABC$ have a ratio of 2:3:4. Which of the following triangles is similar to $\triangle ABC$?

(A) $\triangle DEF$ (4:3:2)
(B) $\triangle PQR$ (1:2:3)
(C) $\triangle LMN$ (1:1:1)
(D) $\triangle STW$ (1:1:1)
(E) $\triangle XYZ$ (4:3:2)
(F) $\triangle MRQ$ (3:2:4)

175. If

$$p = \frac{3\sqrt{2}}{\sqrt{2}+1}$$

Which of the following equals $p-4$?

(A) $3\sqrt{2}+2$
(B) 3
(C) 2
(D) $2\sqrt{2}+6$
(E) $\sqrt{3}+2$

176. A coin is tossed five times. What is the probability that the fourth toss is a head?

(A) $\frac{1}{8}$
(B) $\frac{1}{4}$
(C) $\frac{1}{2}$
(D) $\frac{3}{4}$
(E) $\frac{4}{5}$

177. In what proportion must rice at \$0.8 per pound be mixed with rice at \$0.9 per pound so that the resulting mixture costs \$0.825 per pound?

(A) 1 : 3
(B) 1 : 2
(C) 1 : 1
(D) 2 : 1
(E) 3 : 1

178. The following data represent how many cars are owned by each of the 20 families on Pearl Street:

1, 1, 2, 3, 2, 5, 4, 3, 2, 4, 5, 2, 6, 2, 1, 2, 4, 2, 1, 1

What is the probability that a randomly chosen Pearl Street family owns at least 3 cars?
(A) 1/6
(B) 2/5
(C) 9/20
(D) 13/20
(E) 4/5

179. How many three-digit numbers have no even digit and also do not contain zero?

(A) 50
(B) 60
(C) 75
(D) 100
(E) 125

180. A = C, and O = x° = y°. If A = y°/2 and C = y°/2, find x.
181. If 4*p* is equal to 6*q*, then the expression 2*p*−3*q* must be equal to which of the following?

(A) 0
(B) 2
(C) 3
(D) 4
(E) 6

182. In the figure, if *AB*=8, *BC*=6, AC=10, and *CD*=9, then what is the length of *AD*?

(A) 12
(B) 13
(C) 15

(D) 17
(E) 24

183.
If $x > 2$ and $x < 3$, which of the following must be positive?
I. $(x-2)(x-3)$
II. $(2-x)(x-3)$
III. $(2-x)(3-x)$

(A) I only
(B) II only
(C) III only
(D) I and II only
(E) I and III only

184. In the rectangle *ABCD* shown below, *AF* is parallel to *BE*. If *x*=5 and *y*=10, what is the area of triangle *AFD*?

(A) 2.5
(B) 5
(C) 12.5
(D) 50
(E) 50+5*y*

185. If $x^2 + 4x + 3$ is odd, which of the following values of *x* could make that expression odd?

(A) 3
(B) 5
(C) 8
(D) 13
(E) 16

186. Water is poured into an empty cylindrical tank at a constant rate. After 10 minutes, the height of the water has increased by 7 feet. The tank's radius is 10 feet. What is the rate at which the water is being poured in (in cubic feet per minute)?

(A) $\frac{11}{8}$
(B) $\frac{7}{60}$
(C) $\frac{11}{3}$
(D) 11
(E) 70

187. The selling price of 15 items equals the cost price of 20 items. What is the percentage profit earned by the seller on each item?

(A) 15%
(B) 20%
(C) 25%
(D) 33.3%
(E) 40%

188. Removing which of the following values from the set S={1,2,3,4,5,6} would **increase** the average of the set?

(A) 1
(B) 2
(C) 3
(D) 4
(E) 5
(F) 6

189. In a coordinate plane, the point (b,a) is in Quadrant III. If b and a are both coordinates of that point, in which quadrant can the point (a,b) be located?

(A) I only
(B) II only
(C) III only
(D) IV only
(E) Origin

Passage for Questions 190 and 191

Ragwort was unintentionally brought into New Zealand in the late nineteenth century and, like numerous foreign invaders, rapidly became a major nuisance. By the 1920s, the weed was widespread. What compounded the problem was that its spread coincided with sweeping shifts in farming practices, namely a dramatic transition from raising sheep to dairy operations. Ragwort is full of potent and persistent alkaloids: even honey derived from its flowers carries the toxin in a diluted form. Generally, livestock steer clear of areas overrun by ragwort, but they do so once it edges out grass and clover in their pasture. Although sheep can consume it for months without immediate signs of illness, cattle become sick quickly if they ingest it, and fatalities can occur.

190. The passage indicates that the surge of ragwort was especially poorly timed because it

A. occurred alongside and worsened a downturn in farming
B. took place under conditions that allowed ragwort to spread faster than it otherwise would
C. brought about a heightened level of poisonous compounds in the plants
D. prevented the safe production of honey fit for human consumption
E. resulted in effects on livestock that were more severe than they might have been under different circumstances

191. For the next question, consider each choice independently and choose all that apply.

The passage suggests which of the following regarding the difficulties ragwort creates for dairy farmers?

A. Milk from cows that eat ragwort causes sickness in humans who drink it.
B. Ragwort can take over the vegetation that cattle typically consume.
C. Cattle, unlike sheep, lack the ability to distinguish ragwort from suitable fodder.

Passage for Question 192

Although health-inspection standards for catering companies are more rigorous than those for ordinary restaurants, data from the city health department show that more documented instances of food poisoning originated with banquets served by catering services than from individual restaurant meals.

192. Which of the following, if accurate, best clarifies the seeming contradiction stated above?

A. A much higher number of individuals eat in restaurants than attend catered banquets over any specific period.
B. Catering businesses anticipate the exact number of guests and thus are less likely than restaurants to have leftover food, which is a frequent cause of food-borne illness.
C. Many restaurants also offer catering for large events in addition to their usual service for individual diners.

D. Whether food poisoning occurs at a catered banquet is unrelated to whether the meal is served at the caterer's or the client's location.
E. Individuals tend not to link a meal they have eaten to an ensuing illness unless the illness strikes a group of people who communicate with one another.

Passage for Questions 193 and 194

African American newspapers in the 1930s encountered numerous challenges. For example, given that people who bought African American newspapers also tended to buy general-circulation papers, advertisers selling consumer products frequently overlooked African American publications. This discrimination from advertisers did free the Black press from the sway of advertiser interests. It enabled editors to publish more politically charged content than the large national dailies could, as those relied on advertisers' approval of their ideological stance to maintain revenue. Unfortunately, it also pushed the sale price of these Black newspapers considerably higher than that of general-circulation papers. In some cases, up to two-thirds of publication expenses needed to be covered by subscriptions or by contributions from local politicians and other community stakeholders. Moreover, despite their editorial freedom, African American editors often felt obliged to run excessive amounts of sensational stories, sports coverage, and social news to widen their readership.

193. For the following question, consider each option independently and select all that apply.

From the passage, we can infer that if advertisers had more often chosen to run ads in African American newspapers, which of the following could have occurred?
A. The African American press would have devoted even more space to sports and social events than it already did.
B. African American newspapers might have been sold at a lower cost than the large national dailies.
C. African American newspapers might have faced editorial restrictions akin to those imposed on the big national papers.

194. The author of the passage implies which of the following about the "advertisers" mentioned?

A. They operated under the assumption that placing ads in African American papers would not significantly boost their sales.
B. They failed to accurately gauge the circulation numbers of African American papers.
C. They overlooked the fact that African Americans were also newspaper readers when deciding on ad placements.

D. They stayed away from African American newspapers partly in response to the sensational content of those publications.
E. They attempted to persuade African American publishers to drop their advertising prices.

Passage for Question 195

Some time ago, people in Frieland began paying an energy tax of two Frieland pennies for every unit of energy produced by nonrenewable sources that they used. Following this tax's introduction, the total yearly use of energy from nonrenewable sources steadily declined.

195. If the statements above hold true, which of the following must logically follow from them?

A. Revenues from Frieland's energy tax steadily diminished each year.
B. The total volume of energy consumed in Frieland declined steadily each year.
C. The usage of renewable energy sources in Frieland rose on a consistent basis.
D. The money earned from the energy tax was allocated toward advancing the adoption of renewable energy.
E. Renewable energy usage in Frieland increased considerably in comparison with nonrenewable energy usage.

Passage for Questions 196 to 198

In a plausible, though speculative, scenario, oceanographer Douglas Martinson proposes that temperature increases triggered by global warming might not seriously compromise the stability of Antarctica's environment, where sea ice grows around the continent in autumn and winter and mostly retreats in summer. Certainly, because of higher temperatures, less sea ice might develop during the winter. However, Martinson contends that a warmer atmosphere's impact could be counterbalanced by the following mechanism: sea-ice formation raises surface-water salt levels; if less sea ice develops, there is a reduced bump in salinity. With a smaller increase in surface-water salinity, those waters become less dense and thus are less prone to sink and stir up deeper water. Since the deeper water stores a considerable amount of heat, it would ascend more slowly. Consequently, although there might be a reduction in winter sea-ice coverage, surface waters would stay sufficiently cold so that this reduction would not be drastic.

196. Which of the following is suggested by the passage about present-day Antarctic surface waters?

A. They are more vulnerable to yearly changes in air temperature than they would be if they contained lower salt levels.
B. They contain less salt than they would if global warming were under way.

C. They are more inclined to descend and bring deep water to the surface than they would be if atmospheric temperatures were to rise.
D. They mitigate some of the repercussions of global warming extending beyond Antarctica.
E. They are less influenced by the temperature of deep waters than they would be if atmospheric temperatures rose further.

197. According to the passage, Martinson's view of deep Antarctic waters is that

A. they move to the surface more rapidly than they would if global warming were to happen
B. they hold heat that will amplify the influence of warming air temperatures
C. they would be notably warmed by a rise in atmospheric temperatures
D. they would be saltier than they are now if global warming took effect
E. they are harder to stir up when surface waters have a higher salt concentration than when surface waters are relatively less salty

198. Based on the passage, which of the following applies to the sea ice surrounding Antarctica?

A. The volume of ice forming during winter has been on the decline.
B. Most of the ice that emerges in winter persists through the summer.
C. Even slight fluctuations in sea-ice amounts greatly change the temperature of surface waters.
D. Changes in sea-ice coverage caused by global warming would have a major impact on Antarctic environmental stability.
E. Alterations in sea-ice coverage affect how salty the surface waters become.

Passage for Question 199

Evidence that letting natural sunlight into a store can boost sales emerges from the experience of the only Savefast department store that has a sizable skylight. Sunlight streams into half of the store, reducing the need for electric lighting, while the remaining section relies exclusively on artificial light. Since opening two years prior, the departments situated in the sunlit section have generated notably higher sales than those in the artificially lit section.

199. Which of the following, if true, lends the strongest support to the above claim?

A. On days with heavy cloud cover, more electric lighting is employed in the part of the store beneath the skylight.
B. When the store remains open after sundown, the departments under the skylight do not outsell other departments.
C. Many customers buy products from departments in both sections of the store in a single trip.

D. In addition to the skylight, there are several major architectural contrasts between the two parts of the store.
E. The departments housed under the skylight typically generate the most revenue in other Savefast stores as well.

Passage for Questions 200 to 202

While the elite sixteenth-century Renaissance scholars mastered ancient Roman classics in their original Latin and were able to understand them in the genuine historical context, the majority of their educated peers encountered these classics only via classroom lessons on selected Latin excerpts. These texts were chosen painstakingly by Renaissance teachers, since works composed by and for worldly adult Romans did not always align with the moral lessons Renaissance educators wished to impart; sometimes, they even recommended the opposite. Consequently, teachers put students' needs ahead of textual and historical precision, fragmenting potentially "dangerous" passages into short chunks, using them spontaneously to teach subjects ranging from grammar to science. Therefore, I argue that a reader today cannot definitively know what significance any specific line of Roman poetry or prose might have held for any given educated person of the sixteenth century.

200. The passage primarily intends to discuss

A. the inappropriateness of Roman classics for imparting moral teachings
B. the method by which top sixteenth-century scholars absorbed the Roman classics
C. the impact of Roman classics on the education of Renaissance readers
D. how the Roman classics were taught in the sixteenth century
E. a comparison between Renaissance-era and modern approaches to teaching the Roman classics

201. The text suggests that if a student learned Roman classics under a "typical" sixteenth-century instructor, the probable outcome would be that

A. the student connects a piece of Roman verse to a point about grammar
B. the student argues that a Roman poem focusing on overindulgence is harmless when considered in the original Roman context
C. the student has no difficulty articulating ideas in Latin
D. the student attains comprehensive mastery over extensive portions of the classics
E. the student develops an advanced grasp of Roman poetry but knows very little about Roman prose

202. Which of the following, if valid, would most directly undermine the statement in the passage regarding what today's reader cannot ascertain?

A. Certain current readers have thoroughly studied ancient Roman literature because they majored in classics or have advanced degrees in the field.
B. Some present-day readers have figured out exactly which works of Roman literature were introduced to sixteenth-century students.
C. Scholars now can, with effort, uncover that sixteenth-century instructors used certain seemingly "hazardous" classical works while omitting those that seemed "safe."
D. Many of the classical materials employed by sixteenth-century teachers still exist, complete with marginal notes detailing the lessons that were taught orally from those texts.
E. Several writings by the most acclaimed sixteenth-century Renaissance scholars have been translated from Latin and are accessible to modern readers.

Passage for Questions 203 and 204

In humans, the pilomotor reflex triggers what we call goose bumps. This reaction is widely believed to be vestigial—something that once conferred a greater physiological advantage than it does currently. It occurs when the tiny muscle at the base of each hair follicle contracts, causing the hair to stand up. In animals with feathers, fur, or quills, the result is either a layer of insulating warm air or a more daunting appearance to discourage predators. But in humans, body hair is too minimal to accomplish these tasks. Goose bumps in people might, however, have taken on a new function. Similar to flushing—another mechanism that regulates heat—goose bumps have become linked to emotional reactions, such as fear, anger, or the enjoyment we experience when hearing wonderful music. Consequently, they may serve as a social signal.

203. When discussing this "new function" that goose bumps could have for humans, the author presumes which of the following?

A. A person's emotional responses can be initiated by bodily processes that regulate temperature.
B. The visibility of emotional states to other people has some form of utility.
C. If human body hair were thicker, goose bumps would not have gained an additional function.
D. Animals with fur, feathers, or quills might also experience goose bumps tied to emotion.
E. In human evolution, goose bumps are an older feature than flushing.

204. Which choice best describes the central purpose of the sentence before the last one ("Like . . . music")?

A. It draws a distinction between two different physiological processes.
B. It challenges a widely held misunderstanding about the function of goose bumps in humans.
C. It offers possible explanations for why goose bumps and emotional reactions might be related in humans.
D. It suggests flushing and goose bumps convey the very same emotional state.
E. It provides insight into a potential role goose bumps play in humans.

Passage for Questions 205 to 208

Frederick Douglass was unquestionably the most well-known African American figure of the nineteenth century; when he passed away in 1895, he was among the most prominent public personalities in the United States. In his analysis of Douglass' career as a key abolitionist and advocate for Black rights, Waldo Martin has ignited debate by arguing that Douglass should also occupy a notable position in American intellectual history because he reflected so many strains of nineteenth-century thinking: romanticism, idealism, individualism, liberal humanism, and an unwavering faith in progress. However, this claim itself furnishes support to those who argue that most of Douglass' ideas, precisely because they so typify their era, are now outdated. Douglass' vision of a future "composite American nationality" into which all racial and ethnic differences would merge appears, from the vantage of contemporary pluralist thinkers, not only unrealistic but also fundamentally misguided. Yet one central facet of Douglass' thought seems anything but old-fashioned or irrelevant to our modern concerns: he was unmatched in the nineteenth-century United States for being a persistent and potent critic of the notion of inherent racial inequality. He did not merely repudiate such racist ideas in his orations and writings—he presented his own accomplishments and life story as living proof that proponents of racial hierarchy were mistaken to claim one race could be inherently superior to another.

While Martin underscores Douglass' egalitarian stance against racism, he does not sufficiently elucidate how Douglass' antiracist position meshes with his enthusiastic adoption of the liberal Victorian ideals many of today's thinkers dismiss as naïve or antiquated. In reality, Douglass found those democratic and capitalist principles of his time appealing because they served well in attacking slavery and the White supremacist ideology. One of his go-to rhetorical maneuvers was to reveal the hypocrisy of individuals who professed devotion to democracy and equal opportunity yet still condoned slavery and racial bias. It would have been peculiar had Douglass *not* embraced the liberal optimism of his era, given it proved so valuable in the campaign for racial justice during the national emergency that ultimately led to the end of slavery and the establishment of citizenship rights for African Americans. Though these points might appear obvious, if Martin had given them more attention, he could have more effectively countered those critics who dismiss Douglass' worldview as an obsolete relic. Once one acknowledges that Douglass' foremost commitment was to Black equality—and that he capitalized on the liberal ideals of his day as "weapons" in achieving that end—criticizing him for choosing the best tools available at the time becomes rather difficult.

205. The passage in its entirety can best be described as

A. explaining Douglass' rise as a pivotal abolitionist
B. tracing how Douglass' views originated in nineteenth-century romantic, idealistic, and liberal-humanist thought
C. analyzing Douglass' works and speeches through a modern pluralist lens
D. faulting Martin for overlooking inconsistencies between Douglass' principles and prevailing liberal Victorian ideas
E. offering a reply to those who see Douglass' political ideas as no longer relevant

206. We can deduce that the "present-day intellectuals" hold that

A. Though Douglass employed democratic-capitalist ideas to contest slavery and racism, he did not believe in them sincerely
B. seeing Douglass as representative of his time's intellectual currents is itself an outdated viewpoint
C. Douglass' stance against the idea of innate racial inequality no longer matters to contemporary dialogues
D. Douglass' dedication to Black rights does not provide a satisfactory explanation for his seemingly uncritical acceptance of liberal Victorian ideals
E. Douglass' aspiration to eradicate all racial and ethnic distinctions is neither realistic nor desirable

207. Per the passage, Douglass utilized which of the following to refute the doctrine that there is an inherent racial hierarchy?

A. The narrative of his own life
B. His dream of a merged American nationality
C. The hypocrisy of those who declared themselves liberal idealists
D. The unavoidable end of slavery in the United States
E. The fact that the majority of respected intellectuals favored the abolition of slavery

208. Each of the following elements is cited in the passage as part of Douglass' ideological framework EXCEPT

A. idealism
B. egalitarianism
C. capitalism
D. pluralism
E. humanism

Passage for Question 209

The scarlet gilia plant can produce either red or white blossoms. It had long been theorized that hummingbirds, which feed by day, pollinate its red flowers, whereas hawkmoths, which feed at night, handle pollination of its white flowers. In a recent attempt to confirm this color-based pollination theory, researchers covered some scarlet gilia blooms only overnight, and covered others only during the daytime. Those red flowers that were covered overnight still got pollinated; those white flowers that were covered by day also ended up pollinated.

209. Which of the following, if established, would serve as additional proof indicating that hummingbirds favor the red blossoms and hawkmoths prefer the white blossoms of the scarlet gilia?

A. Scarlet gilia blooms that remained uncovered, whether red or white, were pollinated at roughly the same pace.
B. A subset of red scarlet gilia blooms left uncovered the entire time never ended up pollinated at all.
C. White scarlet gilia blooms covered at night were pollinated at a greater rate than similar white blooms left uncovered.
D. Scarlet gilia plants with red blooms that were covered by day and white blooms that were covered by night did not get pollinated.
E. In late August, once most hummingbirds had migrated but hawkmoths were still abundant, red scarlet gilia plants produced seeds more often than they had earlier in the year.

---

210. The state leader has long been fixated on cutting out the press from the relationship between politicians and the public. This has been the single unifying goal of her seemingly unconnected pursuits since she began her career in government: a resolve to **(i)** ______, and ultimately **(ii)** ______, the media's hold over political communication.

Blank (i) Options
A. conceal

B. erode
C. rejuvenate

Blank (ii) Options
D. augment
E. consolidate
F. end

211. It seems entirely understandable that many current observers of American culture might **(i)** ______ classical music. In our era, the elevated segment of American musical life has become an overfamiliar form of entertainment, detached from the spirit of modern times. Consequently, failing to pay attention to what major orchestras do may not mean **(ii)** ______ anything substantial. During the final decades of the nineteenth century, however, music was revered as the "queen of the arts." Classical music was at its zenith in the United States, **(iii)** ______ the larger cultural landscape.

Blank (i) Options
A. cooperate
B. reinterpret
C. ignore

Blank (ii) Options
D. sacrifice
E. appreciate
F. malign

Blank (iii) Options
G. antagonistic toward
H. generally rejected by
I. centrally embedded in

212. In her astonishingly inventive prose, she went beyond any other twentieth-century writer in English (perhaps in any language) in **(i)** ______ literary style and conventions, and **(ii)** ______ a multilayered network of meaning.

Blank (i) Options
A. reinventing
B. canonizing
C. stabilizing

Blank (ii) Options

D. undoing
E. overpraising
F. misunderstanding

213. When looking for standards in the sense of moral guidelines of what ought to be—rather than looking for what is ordinary and therefore can be deemed normal—ethical theory that focuses on norms attempts to ______.

A. predict
B. mitigate
C. question
D. dictate
E. personalize

214. Last week's unassailable triumph by the figure-skating duo was particularly **(i)** ______ to their chief competitors, who were performing at their absolute best and privately grumbled about the scoring. Moreover, the fact that the winning pair succeeded even while their rivals were **(ii)** ______ underscores how impressive the victory truly was.

Blank (i) Options

A. unsurprising
B. irksome
C. gratifying

Blank (ii) Options

D. terrific
E. nervous
F. inconsistent

215. Once considered a shocking visual effect, having one performer portray multiple roles in a single scene no longer astonishes the average film enthusiast, because such technological wizardry has become so ______.

A. expensive
B. specialized
C. sinister

D. commonplace
E. unreliable

216. It is a grim yet well-founded reproach of some secondary-school history texts that they often present as **(i)** ______ statements that historians argue fervently about, or that are outright **(ii)** ______ by **(iii)** ______ firsthand documents.

Blank (i) Options
A. factual
B. controversial
C. sensational

Blank (ii) Options
D. resolved
E. corroborated
F. contradicted

Blank (iii) Options
G. dubious
H. incomplete
I. reliable

217. In searching for authoritative standards—rather than norms in the sense of the average—this branch of moral philosophy aims to ______.

A. predict
B. mitigate
C. question
D. dictate
E. personalize

218. Investigators aiming to trace forged documents back to the laser printer that created them are **(i)** ______ the reality that the rotating drums and mirrors inside these machines are slightly flawed and yield unique banding traces. Though these trace patterns are **(ii)** ______ to human sight, they can be **(iii)** ______ and analyzed by specialized software that the investigators have spent the past year developing.

Blank (i) Options
A. exploiting

B. facing
C. manipulating

Blank (ii) Options
D. invisible
E. obvious
F. unappealing

Blank (iii) Options
G. detected
H. implemented
I. generated

219. When she arrived in France from her homeland, she certainly was not the ______ student she eventually portrayed herself to be, given that she had access to significant family funds.

A. naïve
B. precocious
C. impecunious
D. ambitious
E. assiduous

220. The environment in which the concert occurred **(i)** ______ the atmosphere of artistic creativity: the ensemble delivered a refined and poised performance, but the sound, which wafted through the chilly, echo-free high-school auditorium, was unexpectedly **(ii)** ______, considering the vigor the musicians appeared to pour into their playing.

Blank (i) Options
A. exacted a toll on
B. encouraged nervousness in
C. solved a dilemma for

Blank (ii) Options
D. clangorous
E. tepid
F. inviting

221. Earlier scholarly examinations often concluded that the public was ______ the manipulative power of mass media. However, one contemporary investigation suggests that, on the contrary, large-scale media seldom bring about significant shifts in social attitudes or behavior.

A. unaware of
B. scornful of
C. susceptible to
D. unimpressed by
E. coping with

222. Commentators have noted that the media once depicted the governor as anything but ineffective; now they cast her as the embodiment of ______.

A. fecklessness
B. brilliance
C. dynamism
D. egoism
E. punctiliousness

223. This composer has never pursued wide appeal: her harsh brand of modernism appears to challenge rather than to ______ the listener.

A. ignore
B. discount
C. woo
D. teach
E. cow

224. The reason that minimum temperatures are climbing more swiftly than maximum ones may connect to cloud cover and evaporative cooling. Clouds can cool days by reflecting sunlight while keeping nights warmer by **(i)** ______ the escape of Earth's heat. Also, additional soil moisture from more frequent precipitation and overcast skies can **(ii)** ______ daytime temperature increases because part of the incoming solar energy is **(iii)** ______ evaporating that moisture.

Blank (i) Options
A. inhibiting

B. exacerbating
C. replicating

Blank (ii) Options
D. augment
E. mask
F. restrain

Blank (iii) Options
G. intensified by
H. unrelated to
I. used up in

225. In a more recent study of the Renaissance, by indicating how that period's artistic bloom was **(i)** ______ bound to its commercial vigor, the author shows that acquisitiveness may be **(ii)** ______ artistic flourishing.

Blank (i) Options
A. questionably
B. intimately
C. skeptically

Blank (ii) Options
D. threatened by
E. inseparable from
F. comparable to

226. Instant fame is often **(i)** ______, especially if there is no **(ii)** ______ to sustain the public's interest—no theatrical or cinematic hits, no notable publications, no remarkable achievements. People quickly lose interest under such circumstances.

Blank (i) Options
A. a fleeting
B. an incomparable
C. an untapped

Blank (ii) Options
D. competing attraction

E. continuity of exposure
F. real achievement

227. We have yet to **(i)** ______ the evaluation of Canada's biodiversity. Although most vertebrates have been examined, the major challenge is the assessment of invertebrates and plant species. This task is **(ii)** ______ not just due to the sheer number of these species but also their variety, as each one calls for a distinct approach.

Blank (i) Options
A. initiate
B. complete
C. limit

Blank (ii) Options
D. repetitious
E. trivial
F. daunting

228. Female labor made a crucial contribution to the growth of European textile manufacturing in the eighteenth century, yet it remains difficult to **(i)** ______. Even though there have been significant **(ii)** ______ in research on women, most analyses of European industrialization still conspicuously omit the role of women's work. Women vastly outnumbered men in textile work, yet data about wages and discussions about growth or living costs **(iii)** ______ regarding male labor alone.

Blank (i) Options
A. track
B. overestimate
C. ignore

Blank (ii) Options
D. advances
E. gaps
F. disinterest

Blank (iii) Options
G. incorporate data only
H. suppress most information
I. too rarely talk

229. The gaps in present-day accounts of the dramatist's life are not **(i)** ______, because much of the documentary foundation on which historians used to rely is **(ii)** ______.

Blank (i) Options

A. abstruse

B. adverse

C. hortatory

Blank (ii) Options

D. credible

E. extant

F. incomplete

230. The firm's attempts to upgrade its safety standards apparently were **(i)** ______, at least if the company's own figures are accurate, indicating that the **(ii)** ______ of incidents that might result in a grave accident went down significantly. Still, independent experts maintain that those statistics are **(iii)** ______. These analysts say that the company has consistently understated both how likely accidents are and how severe they might be in the delicate and poorly understood environment where the firm operates.

Blank (i) Options

A. innovative

B. successful

C. frustrated

Blank (ii) Options

D. frequency of

E. impediments to

F. attention to

Blank (iii) Options

G. deceptive

H. testable

I. consistent

231. The once widespread presumption that mass culture is intrinsically inferior to "high" art is said to have been overturned by academics who seriously study popular media. Nevertheless, this supposed change in perspective might be a bit **(i)** ______.

While scrutinizing popular culture is now acceptable in scholarly circles, the fact that numerous intellectuals feel the need to justify their own **(ii)** ______ blockbuster films or commercial fiction perhaps reveals their continued **(iii)** ______ the traditional divide between high and low culture.

Blank (i) Options

A. counterproductive

B. underappreciated

C. overstated

Blank (ii) Options

D. penchant for

E. distaste for

F. indifference to

Blank (iii) Options

G. aversion to

H. investment in

I. misunderstanding of

232. In his earliest dramas, the playwright made physical illness **(i)** ______ to the plot; from that fact, his first reviewers deduced that he had a special liking for **(ii)** ______ themes.

Blank (i) Options

A. a pivotal

B. a nonexistent

C. an obscure

Blank (ii) Options

D. recondite

E. uncomplicated

F. morbid

233. For much of the early nineteenth century, scientific study at the university languished in ______, despite the presence of many prominent figures.

A. a scintillating

B. a pathetic

C. a controversial
D. an incendiary
E. a veracious

234. Chimpanzees have been seen pretending to be injured in order to affect the behavior of others in the group, indicating that the ability to ______ is not exclusive to humans.

A. cooperate
B. instruct
C. conspire
D. dissemble
E. dominate

235. Some analysts worry about consumers' perception that the electronics industry is always on the verge of major breakthroughs; that perception could hurt the industry by making consumers reluctant to buy products they believe will soon be ______.

A. incompatible
B. devalued
C. obsolete
D. ubiquitous
E. everywhere
F. outmoded

236. Mr. Hirsch says he will aim to preserve the foundation's ______support of thinkers, individuals who are going against the trends in a field or an acknowledged set of opinions.

A. iconoclastic
B. integrative
C. doctrinaire
D. heterodox
E. dogmatic
F. synthesizing

237. That people ______ the musical features of birdsongs suggests that despite the vast evolutionary gulf between birds and mammals, songbirds and humans share some common auditory perceptual abilities.

A. mimic
B. recognize
C. relish
D. are confounded by
E. can make out
F. are puzzled by

238. At nearly 450 pages, the novel is: the author does not often resist the temptation to finish off a ______ chapter, section, or even paragraph with some unnecessary flourish.

A. instructive
B. complex
C. prolix
D. educational
E. long-winded
F. explicit

239. In *The Simple Soybean*, the author is much less restrained in his enthusiasm for the bean's medical efficacy than he is in his technical writings, but he still cautions against treating soy as a ______

A. staple
B. supplement
C. herald
D. panacea
E. cure-all
F. harbinger

240. Retrofitted with stabilizing devices, some of which ______ its aesthetics, the bridge has been reopened, no longer prone to excessive swaying but not quite the breathtaking structure it originally was.

A. impair
B. resist
C. improve
D. enhance
E. restore
F. compromise

241. Through its state associations, the American Medical Association ______ who could become a physician and dominated professions like nursing and occupational therapy.

A. commensurate
B. proportionate
C. kindred
D. affiliated
E. imperative
F. voluntary

242. Despite her relaxed and flexible style, Ms. de la Fressange is ______ businesswoman who knows how to market her brand: herself.

A. a ruthless
B. a creative
C. a canny
D. an industrious
E. a shrewd
F. an effective

243. The band's long-standing strategy of laying leisurely explorations atop a steady funk beat has proven to be surprisingly ______: a concert in Cologne from 1972 sounds as if it could have taken place today.

A. fortuitous
B. foresighted
C. prescient
D. popular
E. serendipitous
F. lucrative

244. If researchers can determine exactly what is wrong with people who suffer from this condition, they may be able to suggest drug therapies or other treatments that could ______ the effects of the damage.

A. mitigate
B. exacerbate
C. specify

D. identify
E. ameliorate
F. stabilize

245. The problem of avoiding duplicate names—such as for Internet domain names or for e-mail accounts—is particularly ______ when the name has to fit into a format that allows only a finite number of possibilities.

A. meager
B. acute
C. agreeable
D. severe
E. beneficial
F. productive

246. Britain is attractive to worldwide advertisers because it is ______ market, so there is no need to tailor advertisements for different parts of the country.

A. a global
B. an uncomplicated
C. a vast
D. a homogeneous
E. a uniform
F. an immense

247. Parkin's ______ characterization of the movement as neoscholastic is too accepted without further investigation.

A. cursory
B. detailed
C. perfunctory
D. biased
E. self-evident
F. complete

248. Factory production made an absence of imperfections so blandly commonplace that the______ of hand-produced goods were now cherished where they once might have been shunned.

A. advantages
B. revivals
C. benefits
D. pretensions
E. blemishes
F. defects

249. After people began to make the transition from gathering food to producing food, human societies followed markedly ______ courses; some adopted herding, others took to tillage, and still others stuck to foraging.

A. divergent
B. rural
C. novel
D. unfamiliar
E. disparate
F. quotidian

250. Although cosmic objects have struck Earth since the planet's very formation, humanity has only recently become aware of these events: two centuries ago the idea that objects orbiting the Sun could collide with Earth was widely ______.

A. ridiculed
B. doubted
C. disseminated
D. promulgated
E. marginalized
F. disbelieved

251. In a strong indication of the way the entire party is ______ the candidate with moderate credentials, the outspokenly conservative former mayor of a major city has promised to raise a substantial amount of money for the candidate's campaign.

A. rallying behind
B. incensed over
C. undecided about
D. mortified over
E. embarrassed about
F. coalescing around

252. A recent study suggests that vitamin E supplements, despite widespread belief in their ______, are no better than sugar pills for delaying the onset of the degenerative disease.

A. potential
B. misuse
C. popularity
D. efficacy
E. prevalence
F. usefulness

253. In France, cultural subsidies are ______: producers of just about any film can get an advance from the government against box-office receipts, even though most such loans are never fully repaid.

A. ubiquitous
B. invaluable
C. sporadic
D. scanty
E. questionable
F. omnipresent

254. Torpey's study has turned a seemingly ______topic, the passport, into a fascinating one by making an original contribution to the sociology of the state.

A. ironic
B. banal
C. provocative
D. witty
E. insipid
F. stimulating

255. A and B are centers of two circles that touch each other externally. What is the area of the circle whose diameter is AB ?

(A) 4
(B) 25
(C) 9

(D) 16
(E) 25/4

256. If $(2x + 1)^2 = 100$, then which of the following COULD equal x ?

(A) –11/2
(B) –9/2
(C) 9/2
(D) 11/2
(E) 17/2

257. What is the greatest prime factor of $24(\ )^2(\ )1$?

A)3
(B) 5
(C) 11
(D) 17
(E) 19

258. a, b, c, d, and e are five consecutive integers in increasing order of size. Which one of the following expressions is not odd?

(A) a + b + c
(B) ab + c
(C) ab + d
(D) ac + d
(E) ac + e

259. The number m yields a remainder p when divided by 14 and a remainder q when divided by 7. If p = q + 7, then which of the following could be the value of m ?

(A) 45
(B) 53
(C) 72
(D) 81
(E) 85
(F) 100

260. A bowl contains one marble labeled 0, one marble labeled 1, one marble labeled 2, and one marble labeled 3. The bowl contains no other objects. If two marbles are drawn randomly without replacement, what is the probability that they will add up to 3?

(A) 1/12
(B) 1/8
(C) 1/6
(D) 1/4
(E) 1/3

261. ABC is a right-angled isosceles triangle, and B is the right angle in the triangle. If AC measures $7\sqrt{2}$, then which one of the following would equal the lengths of AB and BC, respectively?

(A) 7, 7
(B) 9, 9
(C) 10, 10
(D) 11, 12
(E) 7, 12

262. The area of the base of a tank is 100 sq. ft. It takes 20 seconds to fill the tank with water poured at a rate of 25 cubic feet per second. What is the height in feet of the rectangular tank?

263. The ratio of the sum of the reciprocals of x and y to the product of the reciprocals of x and y is 1 : 3. What is the sum of the numbers x and y?

(A) 1/3
(B) 1/2
(C) 1
(D) 2
(E) 4

264. The list price of a commodity is the price after a 20% discount on the retail price. The festival discount price on the commodity is the price after a 30% discount on the list price. Customers purchase commodities from stores at a festival discount price. What is the effective discount offered by the stores on the commodity on its retail price?

(A) 20%
(B) 30%

(C) 44%
(D) 50%
(E) 56%

265. A survey of n people in the town of Eros found that 50% of them prefer Brand A. Another survey of 100 people in the town of Angie found that 60% prefer Brand A. In total, 55% of all the people surveyed together prefer Brand A. What is the total number of people surveyed?

(A) 50
(B) 100
(C) 150
(D) 200
(E) 250

266. If $x + y = 750$, then which of the following additional details alone will determine the numeric value of x ?

(A) $x + 2y = d$
(B) $2x + 4y = 2d$
(C) $2x + 2y = 1500$
(D) $3x = 2250 - 3y$
(E) $2x + y = 15$
(F) $x + 2y = 2235$

267. If n is a positive integer, which of the following numbers must have a remainder of 3 when divided by any one of the numbers 4, 5, and 6?

(A) $12n + 3$
(B) $24n + 3$
(C) $60n + 3$
(D) $80n + 2$
(E) $120n + 3$

268. What is the maximum number of 3 x 3 squares that can be formed from the squares in the 6 x 6 checker board shown?

(A) 4
(B) 6
(C) 12
(D) 16
(E) 24

269. The sum of the first n terms of an arithmetic series whose nth term is n can be calculated by the formula n(n + 1)/2. Which one of the following equals the sum of the first eight terms in a series whose nth term is 2n ?

(A) 24
(B) 48
(C) 56
(D) 72
(E) 96

270. If p = 216^(–1/3) + 243^(–2/5) + 256^(–1/4), then which of the following is an integer?

(A) p/19
(B) p/36
(C) p
(D) 19/p
(E) 36/p
(F) 19p
(G) 36p

271. In a series of five consecutive even integers with middle integer n, the difference between the greatest integer and the smallest integer in the series is

(A) n – 5
(B) 8 if the order is increasing and 10 if the order is decreasing.
(C) 8 if the order is decreasing and 10 if the order is increasing.
(D) 8 whether the order is decreasing or increasing.
(E) 8 whether the integers are positive or negative.

272. There are 750 male and female participants in a meeting. Half the female participants and one-quarter of the male participants are Democrats. How many participants could be both female and Democrat?

(A) 75
(B) 100
(C) 125
(D) 175
(E) 225

273. In the rectangular coordinate, ABCD is a parallelogram. If the coordinates of the points A, B, C, and D are (0, 2), (a, b), (a, 2), and (0, 0), respectively, then b = ?

Points:
A (0, 2) B (a, b) C (a, 2) D (0, 0)

(Enter the numerical value.)

274. If 273m27^{3^m}273m and 4m>14^m > 14m>1, then what is the value of m?

(A) –1
(B) –1/4
(C) 0
(D) 1/4
(E) 1

275. If each of the three nonzero numbers a, b, and c is divisible by 3, then abc must be divisible by which of the following numbers?

(A) 9
(B) 27
(C) 81
(D) 121
(E) 159 304

276. If x + 3 is positive, then which one of the following must be positive?

(A) x – 3
(B) (x – 3)(x – 4)
(C) (x – 3)(x + 3)
(D) (x – 3)(x + 4)
(E) (x + 3)(x + 6)

277. In a market, a dozen eggs cost as much as a pound of rice, and a half-liter of kerosene costs as much as 8 eggs. If the cost of each pound of rice is $0.33, then how many cents does a liter of kerosene cost?

(A) 0.33
(B) 0.44
(C) 0.55
(D) 44
(E) 55

278. If a, b, and c are three different numbers and ax : by : cz = 1 : 2 : –3, then find ax + by + cz.

(A) 0
(B) 1/2
(C) 3
(D) 6
(E) 9

279. If b equals 10% of a and c equals 20% of b, then which of the following equals 30% of c?

(A) 0.0006% of a
(B) 0.006% of a
(C) 0.06% of a
(D) 0.6% of a
(E) 6% of b

280. The remainder when m + n is divided by 12 is 8, and the remainder when m – n is divided by 12 is 6. If m > n, what is the remainder when mn is divided by 6?

(Enter the numerical answer.)

281. In film studies—a visually oriented discipline that is marked by backlit close-ups, eyeline matches, and voyeuristic gazes—scholars have often been tone-deaf to the sounds of music.

A. fixated on
B. obsessed with
C. unconcerned with
D. amused by

E. both red by
F. indifferent to

282. By recognizing commonalities among all the major political parties and by promoting a collaborative decision-making process, the prime minister has made good on his promise to cultivate a leadership style that emphasizes
A. growth
B. politics
C. ideology
D. cooperation
E. differentiation

The following question is based on this passage:

What makes a worker ant perform one particular task rather than another? From the 1970s to the mid-1980s, researchers emphasized internal factors within individual ants, such as polymorphism—the presence in the nest of workers of different shapes and sizes, each suited to a particular task. Other elements then considered to have primary influence upon an ant's career were its age—it might change tasks as it got older—and its genetics. However, subsequent ant researchers have focused on external prompts for behavior. In advocating this approach, Deborah Gordon cites experiments in which intervention in a colony's makeup perturbed worker activity. By removing workers or otherwise altering the nest conditions, researchers were able to change the tasks performed by individual workers.

283. According to the passage, which of the following factors were considered from the 1970s to the mid-1980s to influence the division of labor among a colony's worker ants?
A. Ants' inherited traits
B. The age of the ants
C. The ants' experiences outside the nest

The following question is based on the below passage:

During the 1920s, most advocates of scientific management—Frederick Taylor's method for maximizing workers' productivity by rigorously routinizing their jobs—opposed the five-day workweek. Although scientific managers conceded that reducing hours might provide an incentive to workers, in practice they more often used pay differentials to encourage higher productivity. Those reformers who wished to embrace both scientific management and reduced hours had to make a largely negative case, portraying the latter as an antidote to the rigors of the former. In contrast to the scientific managers, Henry Ford claimed that shorter hours led to greater productivity and profits. However, few employers matched either Ford's vision or his specific interest in mass marketing a product—automobiles—that required leisure for its use, and few unions succeeded in securing shorter hours through bargaining. At its 1928 convention, the American Federation of Labor (AFL) boasted of approximately 165,000 members working five-day, 40-hour weeks. But although this represented an increase of about 75,000 since 1926, about 70 percent of the total came from five extremely well-organized building trades' unions.

284. The passage is primarily concerned with discussing which of the following?

A. The relative merits of two points of view regarding a controversy

B. The potential benefits to workers in the 1920s of a change in employers' policies

C. The reasons for a labor-management disagreement during the 1920s

D. The status of a contested labor issue during the 1920s

E. The role of labor unions in bringing about a reform

285. That the artist chose to remain in his hometown does not mean that he remained (i) ______; on the contrary, he (ii) ______ movements of his day.

Blank (i)

A. provincial

B. capricious

C. obstinate

Blank (ii)

D. knew nothing about

E. made light of

F. kept abreast of

286. The lizards snapped up insects that are so (i) ______ that other potential predators avoid them. Among the lizards' prey were some beetles that they initially (ii) ______ because the insects were spraying their hot, irritant defense chemical at the time. Yet even these produced no apparent ill effects, since the lizards, having eaten, proceeded on their way (iii) ______ enough.

Blank (i)

A. rare

B. nutritious

C. noxious

Blank (ii)

(Answer choices for Blank (ii) are provided in the answer key.)

Blank (iii)

(Answer choices for Blank (iii) are provided in the answer key.)

The following question is based on this passage

This passage is adapted from material published in 2001. In 1998 scientists using the neutrino detector in Kamioka, Japan, were able to observe several thousand neutrinos—elusive, tiny subatomic particles moving at nearly the speed of light and passing through almost everything in their path. The Kamioka findings have potentially far-reaching ramifications. They strongly suggest that the neutrino has mass, albeit an infinitesimal amount. Even a tiny mass means that neutrinos would outweigh all the universe's visible matter, because of their vast numbers. The findings also suggest that a given neutrino does not have one stable mass or one stable identity; instead it oscillates from one identity or "flavor" (physicists' term describing how neutrinos interact with other particles) to another. This oscillation may explain why, although the Sun is a large source of neutrinos, detectors capture far fewer solar neutrinos than the best theory of solar physics predicts: the neutrinos may be changing to flavors undetectable by detectors. Finally, while the standard particle-physics model—which describes all matter in terms of twelve fundamental particles and four fundamental forces—does not allow for neutrinos with mass, there are theories that do. Further experiments to confirm that neutrinos have mass could help physicists determine which, if any, of these theories is correct.

287. The primary purpose of the passage is to

A. evaluate the merits of a particular theory in light of new evidence

B. discuss scientists' inability to account for certain unexpected discoveries

C. point out certain shortcomings in a long-standing theory

D. compare several alternative explanations for a particular phenomenon

E. consider some implications of certain scientific findings

288. Although the compound is abundant in the environment at large, its presence in the air is not _______; only in the form of underwater sediment does it cause damage.

A. trivial

B. detectable

C. deleterious

D. substantial

E. detrimental

F. inconsequential

289. Bureaucrats tend to (i) _______ on matters of authority. So it is surprising that the European Commission is proposing to hand back some of its antitrust powers to national governments. Such a willingness to (ii) _______ power is quite (iii) _______. Perhaps the commission, so often a byword for meddling, bungling, and even corruption, is starting to put its house in order following the forced resignation of the previous lot of commissioners last year.

Blank (i)

A. value complex procedures

B. guard their authority jealously

C. shirk many of their responsibilities

Blank (ii)

D. devolve

E. misuse

F. appropriate

Blank (iii)

G. troubling

H. encouraging

I. predictable

290. It can be inferred from the passage that Gordon and earlier researchers would agree with which of the following statements about worker ants?

A. Disruption of the nest can affect workers' roles.

B. Genetics predominates over other factors in determining a worker ant's role.

C. An individual worker's tasks can change during its lifetime.

The following questions is based on this passage:

In November 1753, the British author Sarah Fielding accepted half the payment for her novel The Cry and asked that the other half, when due, go to her "or to whomsoever I shall appoint," perhaps indicating that the remaining share was intended for someone else. Indeed, many think that the novel was a collaborative venture between Fielding and Jane Collier. This particular collaboration was likely enough, as the two were close friends with common interests. They wrote jointly authored letters, were both published authors with a lively interest in each other's work, and were enthusiastic supporters of didacticism and innovation in fiction—central concerns of The Cry. However, contemporaries ascribed the work solely to Fielding, and there is nothing in the novel that is incompatible with Fielding's other writings.

291. The passage presents which of the following as evidence in favor of Fielding and Collier's having collaborated in writing *The Cry*?

A. Their friendship

B. Their joint authorship of correspondence

C. Their approach to fiction

292. In his unexpurgated autobiography, Mark Twain commented freely on the flaws and foibles of his country, making some observations so _______ that his heirs and editors feared they would damage Twain's reputation if not withheld.

A. buoyant

B. acerbic

C. premonitory

D. laudatory
E. temperate

293. According to the passage, one significant implication of the discovery that neutrinos have mass is that such a discovery would

A. cast doubt on the solar origins of many of the neutrinos that reach Earth
B. help to establish the validity of the standard particle-physics model
C. indicate that most of the visible matter of the universe is composed of neutrinos
D. entail that the total weight of all the visible matter in the universe is less than that of all the neutrinos in the universe
E. mean that the speed with which neutrinos normally move can be slowed by certain types of matter

294. An innovation of the eighteenth-century cookbook writer Mary Cole was that in her work she (i) _______ the earlier books from which her recipes were drawn. Even in those numerous instances in which she had collated into a single version, which she could have called her own, the recipes of several earlier writers, she (ii) _______ them.

Blank (i)
A. preserved
B. enhanced
C. acknowledged

Blank (ii)
D. took pains to cite
E. sought to imitate
F. could not surpass

Based on this passage:

Despite a dramatic increase in the number of people riding bicycles for recreation in Parkville, a recent report by the Parkville Department of Transportation shows that the number of accidents involving bicycles has decreased for the third consecutive year.

295. Which of the following, if true during the last three years, best reconciles the apparent discrepancy in the facts?

A. The Parkville Department of Recreation confiscated abandoned bicycles and sold them at auction to any interested Parkville residents.
B. Increased automobile and bus traffic in Parkville had been the leading cause of the most recent increase in automobile accidents.
C. Because of the local increase in the number of people bicycling for recreation, many out-of-town bicyclists ride in the Parkville area.

D. The Parkville Police Department enforced traffic rules for bicycle riders much more vigorously and began requiring recreational riders to pass a bicycle safety course.

E. The Parkville Department of Transportation canceled a program that required all bicycles to be inspected and registered each year.

296. Consumers may think that genetic engineering of foods is something new, but humans have been modifying plants for ages; the _______ is not that new genes are introduced but that genes can now be moved from one species to another.

A. novelty

B. quandary

C. advantage

D. innovation

E. discrepancy

F. predicated

297. Deacon attempts what seems impossible: a book rich in scientific insights, in a demanding discipline, that nevertheless is accessible to _______.

A. skeptics

B. experts

C. nonspecialists

D. zealots

E. authorities

F. laypersons

298. Despite relying on the well-to-do for commissions, the portrait painter was no _______: he depicted the character of those he painted as he perceived it.

A. hypocrite

B. egotist

C. sycophant

D. adulator

E. braggart

F. coward

Based on this passage:

Mayor: Four years ago, when we reorganized the city police department in order to save money, critics claimed that the reorganization would make the police less responsive to citizens and would thus lead to more crime. The police have compiled theft statistics from the years following the reorganization that show that the critics were wrong. There was an overall decrease in reports of thefts of all kinds, including small thefts.

299. Which of the following, if true, most seriously challenges the mayor's argument?

A. When city police are perceived as unresponsive, victims of theft are less likely to report thefts to the police.

B. The mayor's critics generally agree that police statistics concerning crime reports provide the most reliable available data on crime rates.

C. In other cities where police departments have been similarly reorganized, the numbers of reported thefts have generally risen following reorganization.

D. The mayor's reorganization of the police department failed to save as much money as it was intended to save.

E. During the four years immediately preceding the reorganization, reports of all types of theft had been rising steadily in comparison to reports of other crimes.

ANSWERS

1. A writer who "has a predilection for focusing" on something makes it a significant element in his or her work, so the correct choice for Blank (i) must suggest importance. Among the options, "a pivotal" fits that meaning. Concerning the second blank, since the playwright's early critics noticed this emphasis on disease, it must be something rather grim or disturbing. Thus "morbid" is the right choice.
   Correct Answer: (i) a pivotal (A) and **(ii) morbid (F)**
2. Normative ethics seeks standards of what ought to be done, not merely descriptions of what is. Therefore it aims to *establish or impose* these norms. "Dictate" is the only choice conveying that sense of setting authoritative guidelines.
   Correct Answer: dictate (Choice D)
3. The "although" setup tells us that clouds warm nights by *reducing* heat loss, so Blank (i) must reflect preventing or slowing something. "Inhibiting" works best. Next, the text points out how extra moisture and cloud cover *limit* daytime heating. "Restrain" fits that. Finally, part of the solar energy is *consumed* by evaporation, so "used up in" is correct.
   Correct Answer: (i) inhibiting (A), (ii) restrain (F), (iii) used up in (I)
4. Since the independent analysts consider the company's data to be inaccurate, the third blank must reveal that the statistics are misleading, i.e. "deceptive." With that in mind, in the company's own data, safety efforts appear successful, so Blank (i) is "successful." The specific aspect that was declining must be the "frequency of" incidents.
   Correct Answer: (i) successful (Choice B), (ii) frequency of (Choice D), (iii) deceptive (Choice G)
5. The phrase "despite the presence of numerous luminaries" implies that science at the university was in a negative state. The option "pathetic" suggests a woeful condition, which contrasts with the idea that outstanding thinkers were there but did not uplift the atmosphere enough.
   Correct Answer: a pathetic (Choice B)
6. The question is why a special effect that initially astonished audiences is no longer startling. "Commonplace" captures the idea of such effects becoming so usual that viewers are no longer surprised.
   Correct Answer: commonplace (Choice D)
7. The sentence says the evidence historians use is *not complete*, so the resulting gaps in the accounts can't be small. That means the gaps are not "trifling." Paired with that, the evidence is "incomplete."
   Correct Answer: (i) trifling (A) and (ii) incomplete (F)
8. Researchers are using these printing imperfections to their advantage, so Blank (i) is "exploiting." Since the patterns are not readily visible to the naked eye, they must be

"invisible." But they can be "detected" with computer analysis.

Correct Answer: (i) exploiting (A), (ii) invisible (D), (iii) detected (G)

9. Such book reviews, when at their best, are indeed negative or critical but are written with a constructive motive. So "adverse" best describes them. The author hopes the writer will recognize their "transgressions" and make improvements.

   Correct Answer: (i) adverse (B) and (ii) transgressions (E)

10. Since Jardine showed a very close relationship between the era's artistic flowering and its commercial vitality, the terms describing that link must suggest closeness. So "intimately" and "inseparable from" are the matching ideas.

    Correct Answer: (i) intimately (B), (ii) inseparable from (E)

11. The winning pair's rivals felt the outcome was not deserved and complained about the judging, indicating the victory annoyed them, i.e. "irksome." Then, noting the rivals were also impressive, the second blank describing the rivals must be "terrific."

    Correct Answer: (i) irksome (B) and (ii) terrific (D)

12. Since the student actually had considerable family wealth, she was *not* penniless. Thus the idea that she later presented herself as "impecunious" was false.

    Correct Answer: impecunious (Choice C)

13. The text stresses how the role of women, though extensive, has been neglected in historical data, making it difficult to *measure or follow* female labor precisely. So "track" fits Blank (i). The field of women's studies has made "advances," but the economic analyses *still* focus only on men's data. They "incorporate data only" on the male labor force.

    Correct Answer: (i) track (A), (ii) advances (D), (iii) incorporate data only (G)

14. The supposed collapse of the high/low culture distinction may be exaggerated—thus "overstated." Many intellectuals still feel a need to justify their "penchant for" popular culture. This reveals continued "investment in" the old hierarchy.

    Correct Answer: (i) overstated (C), (ii) penchant for (D), (iii) investment in (H)

15. The passage emphasizes how far this writer went in breaking new ground. She was "reinventing" language, "undoing" stylistic rules, and "introducing" a fresh structural complexity.

    Correct Answer: (i) reinventing (A), (ii) undoing (D), (iii) introducing (I)

16. The auditorium acoustics imposed a negative influence, so we say the venue "exacted a toll." Consequently, despite the performers' energetic, polished playing, the sound itself was "tepid."

    Correct Answer: (i) exacted a toll (A), (ii) tepid (E)

17. These days, classical music might be taken as formulaic and disconnected, so it's understandable if students "ignore" it. Missing out on it is not a great "sacrifice," given its perceived stagnation. In the late Gilded Age, though, classical music was "centrally

embedded in" the broader culture.

Correct Answer: (i) ignore (C), (ii) sacrifice (D), (iii) centrally embedded in (I)

18. The composer's stark modernism runs counter to courting popularity. Hence she does not try to "woo" the audience. This contrasts sharply with defying them.

Correct Answer: woo (Choice C)

19. The textbooks are criticized for presenting certain claims as fact even though historians vigorously contest or outright contradict them. So (i) must be "factual." Next, if they're contradicted, that rules out "resolved" or "corroborated." They're "contradicted" by a "reliable" source.

Correct Answer: (i) factual (A), (ii) contradicted (F), (iii) reliable (I)

20. The sentence implies Canada's biodiversity study has not been finished—thus "complete" fits Blank (i). Assessing all the invertebrates and plants would be "daunting," given the scale and variability of species.

Correct Answer: (i) complete (B), (ii) daunting (F)

21. The observed chimpanzee behavior—pretending to be hurt—requires the capacity to *deceive.* Only "dissemble" involves presenting a false appearance to influence others.

Correct Answer: dissemble (Choice D)

22. The older studies cited believed the public *was* strongly affected by mass communications. The new study refutes that. The only answer that implies people were strongly influenced is "susceptible to."

Correct Answer: susceptible to (Choice C)

23. The media's old portrayal was of a highly capable governor, so the new portrayal is the opposite—someone incompetent. Of the choices, "fecklessness" captures that sense of ineffectiveness.

Correct Answer: fecklessness (Choice A)

24. If no follow-up or genuine achievement keeps the public interested, fame quickly fades. So "a fleeting" best fits the notion of short-lived celebrity. Also, there needs to be "real achievement" to retain the public's attention.

Correct Answer: (i) a fleeting (A), (ii) real achievement (F)

25. The governor's entire career focus has been on cutting out the media as a go-between. This suggests her first step is to "erode" that influence, with the ultimate goal to "end" it altogether.

Correct Answer: (i) erode (B), (ii) end (F)

26. The proper pair of words that complete the sentence are:

- **D. exacerbated**
- **F. worsened**

Rationale: The sentence implies that the involvement of foreign technocrats made the country's problems more severe, hence "exacerbated" and "worsened" both convey the idea of making the issues worse.

27. The passage shows that Glass's work reflects:

- **A. A return to the use of popular music in classical compositions**
- **C. A long-standing tendency to incorporate elements from two apparently disparate musical styles**

Rationale: The passage explains that Glass revived the practice of incorporating popular elements (validating option A), and emphasizes his consistent blend of rock and classical styles (supporting option C). The other option (B) is not supported by the text.

28. The correct completions are:

- **Blank (i): A. overshadowed**
- **Blank (ii): E. obscure**
- **Blank (iii): I. superficiality of our theories**

Rationale: The passage highlights that the author avoids letting political factors diminish (or "overshadow") the facts and does not let those factors "obscure" his thorough presentation. Moreover, the mention of significant gaps in knowledge is best captured by the "superficiality of our theories."

29. The two words that suitably complete the sentence are:

- **C. original**
- **F. innovative**

Rationale: Despite the presence of some pioneering ideas, the overall work is not viewed as fundamentally groundbreaking. "Original" and "innovative" both convey that nuance, while the other options do not fit the context.

30. The correct word for the blank is:

- **B. imperceptibly**

Rationale: The sentence describes a transition from land to ice so gradual that it goes unnoticed, which is best captured by "imperceptibly." The other options do not explain the seamless blending of the terrain.

31. The issue addressed in the passage is:

- **E. Whether it has caused certain of Glass's works to be derivative in quality**

Rationale: The passage explicitly explains that even though Glass uses popular elements, his music remains distinctly his own and is not simply a rehashed version of popular music. Thus, the focus is on dispelling the notion of derivativeness.

32. For Caravaggio's sentence, the best answers are:

- **Blank (i): C. eminence**
- **Blank (ii): D. tumultuous**

Rationale: The sentence implies that as Caravaggio's reputation and status as an artist increased (i.e., his eminence), his life became increasingly disorderly or "tumultuous." The alternatives do not capture this cause-and-effect relationship as clearly.

33. D: None of these statements may be made conclusively. Because you do not know the exact distribution of heights, you cannot be certain that 68% are within that range (that assumes a normal distribution), nor can you know that half the students are taller or shorter than the mean, nor that 1.64 m is the most common single height.

34. C: The systematic error is 2.1 pounds. The reading is consistently off by that amount, so there is no random fluctuation here (the scale is precise but not accurate).

35. D: 0.00150000 has 6 significant digits. In contrast, 1,500,000 has only 2, 1.5000×105 has 5, and 0.15000 has 5.

36. A: 254 mm. An inch is approximately 2.54 cm, which is 25.4 mm or 0.0254 m. The alternatives are off by powers of ten.

37. C: II and III. A neutron decays into a proton plus an electron (beta particle) and a neutrino (often accompanied by gamma radiation). Alpha particles are two protons plus two neutrons and are not produced in beta decay.

38. C: Its nucleon number decreases by four. Emitting an alpha particle (2 protons + 2 neutrons) lowers the atomic number by 2 and the mass number by 4.

39. C: They have the same number of protons, but different numbers of neutrons. That is precisely the definition of isotopes of an element.

40. A: Matter is converted into energy. Einstein's equation E = mc2 implies that mass can be transformed into energy and vice versa.

41. C: fusion reactions. The sun's core fuses hydrogen into helium, releasing enormous amounts of energy.
42. B: The new nucleus is unstable. Absorbing a neutron pushes the nucleus into a less stable state, leading to fission, which increases the average binding energy per nucleon.
43. C: 7.2 × 104 years. Every half-life (2.4 × 104 years) halves the material. After three half-lives, 1/8 remains (which is 12.5%); so 87.5% has decayed. 3×2.4×104 = 7.2×104.
44. A: A 10.2 eV photon is emitted. The first excited state of hydrogen is 10.2 eV above ground. Returning to ground emits a photon of that energy.
45. C: −3.6. Multiplying the three magnifications (3.0 × −4.0 × 0.3) gives −3.6 total.
46. D: A ray that strikes the surface of a lens follows Snell's law for refraction is correct physics, but it is not one of the simplified ray-diagram principles typically listed for a thin lens.
47. B: Chromatic aberration involves different colors refracting differently. Mirrors reflect light, so no refraction-based color dispersion occurs.
48. C: 15 cm. For two thin lenses in contact, 1/f_total = 1/f1 + 1/f2 = 1/30 + 1/30 = 2/30, so f_total = 15 cm.
49. A: 0.39. Magnification is image distance / object distance. 19 ÷ 49 ≈ 0.39.
50. D: 20 cm behind the lens. Using 1/f = 1/o + 1/i with f=10 and o=20 yields i=20 cm (positive sign means behind the lens).
51. C: The image may be right side up or upside down, depending on the location of the object relative to the focal point.
52. C: The image will be smaller and right side up. Convex mirrors always create images that are upright and reduced in size.
53. D: At the focal point. Parallel rays reflect and intersect at the focus of a concave mirror.
54. C: Snell's law places a limit on the angle of refraction. Beyond a certain critical angle, total internal reflection occurs.
55. C: The speed of light in water depends on its wavelength. Different wavelengths refract at different angles, separating sunlight into a spectrum.
56. C: It is below 45°. Because n2 > n1, the refracted angle is always less than the angle of incidence. Increasing the incidence angle from 45° to 50° still yields a refracted angle < 45°.
57. B: For diffuse reflection, the surface irregularities are large compared to the wavelength, so the light scatters in many directions.
58. B: Laser is an acronym from light amplification by stimulated emission of radiation. Lasers produce light because the substance used goes into a relatively stable excited state before emitting light. In phosphorescence, a substance absorbs light and goes into a relatively stable excited state. Light is re-emitted at a later point in time. Radioactivity and blackbody radiation are different phenomena. Hence the best matching phenomenon among those choices is (b) phosphorescence."

59. B: threshold frequency. This is the photoelectric effect concept: light's energy is quantized, so there's a minimum frequency needed to eject electrons.

60. A: Light waves' electromagnetic fields can be oriented in a specific direction, producing polarization.

61. A: The more slits per inch, the closer the lines of destructive interference, producing a sharper separation of maxima and minima.

62. B: Diffraction and interference. The two slits create two wavefronts that combine constructively and destructively.

63. D: The lengths of the paths differ by an integral number of wavelengths, causing the peaks to line up in phase for maximum constructive interference.

64. A: 0 amperes. The average current of an AC waveform over a full cycle is zero, even though the instantaneous current is not zero.

65. B: 5 amperes. $P = IV \Rightarrow I = P / V = 50 \text{ W} / 10 \text{ V} = 5 \text{ A}$.

66. A: Infinite time. A capacitor in an RC circuit discharges exponentially and never fully reaches 0 volts, though it will get close after several time constants.

67. C: 20 μF. Since these capacitors are in parallel, you simply add the capacitance. 5 + 15 = 20 μF.

68. A: 2-microfarads. These are in series, so 1/Ctotal = 1/3 + 1/6 = 1/2 => Ctotal = 2 μF.

69. B: ½CV2. The energy stored in a capacitor is ½C(V2).

70. C: It has remained the same. The capacitance depends only on the geometry and material of the capacitor, not on the battery's voltage.

71. A: The resistance of the two wires is the same. Doubling length and cross-sectional area simultaneously leaves $R = \rho L/A$ unchanged.

72. B: 12 Ω. The 2 and 4 ohm are in series => 6 ohms, which is in parallel with 3 ohms => total 2 ohms. Add that to 10 ohms => 12 ohms total.

73. B: The current flowing in the resistor decreases slightly because of the small additional internal resistance of the ammeter, though ideal ammeters are assumed to have negligible resistance.

74. C: Increasing the current increases the voltage if resistance stays the same. $V = IR$.

75. A: A battery transforms chemical potential energy into electrical energy.

76. D: Watt-volts is not a valid expression of current. (A= coulombs/s, or electrons/s, or V/Ω.)

77. D: Can't be determined from the information given. The two batteries are opposed, and their voltages are not specified.

78. C: UHF radio waves, microwaves, visible light, x-rays. This is the correct ascending frequency order.

79. B: The "color" of light is determined by its frequency, not its wavelength alone. However, in typical usage for visible light in a given medium, wavelength is also used interchangeably. The original official key says answer B is untrue because frequency truly sets color.

80. C: All frequencies of light travel at the same speed in a vacuum, about 3×108 m/s.

81. A: To increase the magnetic field inside the solenoid. More loops concentrate the field lines inside.

82. B: The particle is positively charged, so it's moving in a direction opposite the electron's. They attract magnetically if the currents are in the same direction (electron negative current is to the left, the positive charge's conventional current is also to the left if it physically travels to the right).

83. C: 4.5 × 10−13 newtons. F = qvB sinθ => (1.6×10−19 C)(8×106 m/s)(0.5 T)(sin 45°) ≈ 4.5×10−13 N.

84. B: Gauss's law. The flux through a surface is proportional to the enclosed charge.

85. C: The paper will acquire a positive charge and be repelled by the comb. After initial attraction by induction, contact allows electrons to flow from the paper to the comb, leaving net positive charge on the paper.

86. B: At an infinite distance, the dipole field is effectively zero, so the potential is zero.

87. A: The positive charge will be on the northern side, aligning with the electric field direction from south to north.

88. D: The charges are equal in magnitude and have opposite signs. That's the definition of an electric dipole.

89. B: The potential energy of the electron increases because it's being forced to move in the same direction as the field. The correct answer is that the potential energy of the electron increases if it moves along the field lines—**that typically means it's going from negative plate to positive plate**.

90. B: The charge will be distributed uniformly at the surface of the sphere. Excess charge on a conductor resides on its surface.

91. D: The field is uniform. The diagram indicates equally spaced, parallel lines.

92. D: Greater than 2d. The positive charge is repelled by +2q more strongly and must be placed even farther to the right beyond -q for net force zero.

93. B: A material that contains moveable electric charges. That's the essential property of an electrical conductor.

94. B: The net charge of an isolated system remains constant. Charges can be transferred, but the total is conserved.

95. B: It is an attractive force. The charged object induces an opposite charge on the neutral object.

96. D: Bulk Modulus. It relates changes in volume to changes in pressure for a solid or fluid.

97. B: The average distance between water molecules increases in the crystal structure of ice.

98. A: The elastic limit occurs when the deformation is no longer fully reversible.

99. C: It increases slightly. The high external pressure squeezes the aluminum, reducing its volume and increasing density.

100. D: The fluid does not have any rotating points, whirlpools, or eddies. Irrotational flow means no circulation.

101. C: 16.7 m/s. Using continuity, A1v1 = A2v2 => π(5 cm)2 ×6 = π(3 cm)2 × v2 => v2=16.7 m/s.

102. B: Decrease L, increase r, and decrease η to increase the flow rate, per Poiseuille's law.

103. C: 4.3 ×105 N. The gauge pressure is ρgh=1000×9.8×14=1.37×105. Multiply by πr2=3.14×(1)2=3.14 => ~4.3×105 N.

104. A: 24 N. By Pascal's principle, F/A is the same in each cylinder. The ratio of areas is (2 cm)2 : (24 cm)2 => 1:144 => the force ratio is 1:144. 3500N ÷144≈24N.

105. C: It is equal to the submarine's weight. Constant depth => equilibrium => buoyant force=weight.

106. B: 0.80. The density ratio is 5/4=1.25, so the volume ratio is the inverse=0.80.

107. B: Echolocation. Ultrasound imaging relies on sound reflecting off internal structures.

108. A: 12.5 newtons. The wave speed is 50 m/s => T=μv2 =>0.005×(50)2=12.5.

109. C: 425 Hz. Third harmonic =>1.5 waves in 1.2 m => λ=0.8 => f=340÷0.8=425.

110. A: pitch. Frequency corresponds to perceived pitch in sound.

111. A: It is faster. Lower density => higher speed of sound.

112. B: pressure differential of fluctuations. Loudness is a subjective measure; amplitude is half the difference between condensation and rarefaction.

113. A: Refraction means a change in direction when entering a new medium. The frequency remains the same, though the wavelength and speed change.

114. C: 0.25 seconds. The beat frequency is 504-500=4 Hz => period=1/4=0.25 s.

115. A: 0.1 Hz. The fundamental wave is a half wave in the string => λ=40 => f=4/40=0.1 => or using v=λf =>4=40f =>f=0.1.

116. C: The pendulum will swing higher. Resonance builds amplitude at the resonant frequency.

117. A: 0. Peak meets trough => destructive interference => amplitude sums to zero.

118. B: 36 meters per second. Wave speed=frequency×wavelength=12×3=36.

119. A: I only. Reflected from a receding car => longer wavelength => lower frequency.

120. C: The magnitude of the acceleration is at a maximum at the endpoints (where velocity is zero and the string tension is minimal).

121. C: 1.26 seconds. If the argument is 5.0 t=2π => t=2π/5=>1.26 s.

122. D: 196 newtons per meter. Force=mg=980 => kx=980 => x=5 =>k=980/5=196.

123. D: An angle indicating the wave cycle's instantaneous location. Phase is the fraction of a cycle measured in radians or degrees.

124. B: $3.60. 5 kW×12 h=60 kWh×$0.06=$3.60.

125. D: If a force is conservative, any component of the force is equal to the change in potential energy divided by position. It doesn't matter which path is taken.

126. B: Total energy is conserved in an isolated system. Mechanical energy may be lost to heat, but total energy remains constant.

127. C: Halved. The force is ¼ as large at 2R, while potential is ½ as large, so ratio=1/4 ÷1/2=1/2.

128. D: Four times as much. The spring is stretched twice as far with double the mass => (2x)2=4x2 => 4 times the stored energy.

129. C: 2.5 R. The top requires mg=mv2/r. v2=gR. Then from energy conservation h=½R+2R=2.5R.

130. B: The motorcycle has 8 times the bicycle's kinetic energy, since KE=½mv2 => doubling m and v => factor of 8.

131. A: 2 kilowatts. Average force=1000 N (peak 2000, triangular average). Work=1000N×0.2m=200J over 0.1s =>2000W=2kW.

132. B: The change in kinetic energy of an object is equal to the work done on that object (W=ΔKE).

133. C: A falling object experiences a change in potential energy. Gravitational work depends only on vertical displacement, not path.

134. A: 0 joules. The net force=0 for uniform speed, so no net work. Friction cancels the pulling force.

135. B: 3.1 m/s. By momentum conservation, combined mass 175 => total momentum=548 => v=548/175=3.1.

136. D: More than 10 m/s. It's an elastic collision with a heavier incoming ball, so the smaller ball speeds off faster than 10 m/s.

137. A: The speed of the first car decreases by half. Momentum is conserved => final speed=½ initial if masses latch together.

138. D: The object's impulse increases. Gravity acts continuously, accelerating the ball => momentum grows => impulse accumulates.

139. A: The total momentum is conserved in a closed system, though kinetic energy generally is not.

140. B: II only. Outer space is not negligible gravity; orbit is free-fall. Rolling a baseball is not free fall. A ski jumper is.

141. B: A hollow cylinder has a larger average radius of mass distribution => greater moment of inertia.

142. C: Newton's third law. The expelled air pushes in one direction, the balloon is propelled in the opposite.

143. B: The masses will remain balanced. Halving both distances equally keeps the net torques the same.

144. D: 3048 N is the tension in each wire. With 200 kg => weight=1960N. The wires share the load at sin40 => T=1960/(2×0.64)=1524 => but the original official key gave 1524 N.

145. B: 11.1 N. Acceleration=25/(9kg)=2.78 => tension=4×2.78=11.1.

146. B: 2 m/s2. Net force=98N for a difference of 294N−196N => 98N => total mass=50 =>a=98/50=1.96=>2 m/s2.

147. B: 2. There is one fixed pulley with mechanical advantage 1, and one moveable pulley with advantage 2 => total 2.

148. C: 59 N. Static friction=μs×mg=0.6×(10×9.8)=58.8≈59.

149. C: The maximum speed is 1.4v. Doubling r => max speed grows by √2 for the same banking angle.

150. C: The force of friction between the wall and your body is stronger than gravity, preventing you from slipping.

151. D: Both spheres move slightly towards each other. The gravitational force is the same in magnitude on each, per Newton's 3rd law.

152. A: The force of the table on the box is the reaction to the weight of the box.

153. B: II and III only. A newton is not fundamental; first law can be derived from second; not from universal gravity.

154. A: Pushing a billiard ball on a smooth surface demonstrates Newton's first law (inertia) well, as it continues rolling with no net force.

155. C: III is true. Center of mass moves at a constant speed in a circular orbit. I and II are not necessarily correct.

156. C: The acceleration is -9.8 m/s2. Gravity never turns off or changes sign.

157. B: 2 seconds. Speed changes 10 m/s at 5 m/s2 => 2 s.

158. C: 4 m/s. 400 m /100 s=4.

159. C: Displacement is as low as 5 if the second walk is 180° reversed, up to <13 otherwise.

160. C: Velocity is a vector with both magnitude and direction; distance, speed, and time are scalars.

161. D: 35.59. Summing is 35.5918, but only two decimals are allowed because of 23.04 and 7.12 => 35.59.

162. B: 2.9900 has 5 significant digits. 0.2990 and 2.997 each have 4, and 0.00209 has 3.

163. **(E)**

Let's test values within 1<*p*<31

- If *p*=1.5, then p2=2.25 and 2p=3. Since 2.25<3, I is true.
- If *p*=2, then p2=4 and 2p=4. Since 4=4, II is true.
- If *p*=2.5, then p2=6.25 and 2p=5. Since 6.25>5, III is true.

Since all conditions can be satisfied for some *p*, the correct answer is **(E)**.

164. **(A, B, C, D, E)**

The equation is *x*+2*y*=7.

- If $x = 0$, then $2y = 7 \Rightarrow y = 3.5$.
- If $x = 2$, then $2y = 5 \Rightarrow y = 2.5$.
- If $x = 3$, then $2y = 4 \Rightarrow y = 2$.
- If $x = 5$, then $2y = 2 \Rightarrow y = 1$.
- If $x = 7$, then $2y = 0 \Rightarrow y = 0$.

All choices are possible, so the correct answer is **(A, B, C, D, E)**.

165. (A, B, G)

The largest product is obtained by selecting three numbers farthest from zero while ensuring the result is **positive**.

1. The best choices are −9,−5, 10:

   (−9)×(−5)×10=450

2. Other choices give smaller products.

The correct answer is **(A, B, G)**.

166. (D)

Given *y*=3*x* and *x*=*z*, we substitute *z* for *x*:

y=3*z*, which means *y* is always greater than *z*.

The correct answer is **(D)** ***y*> *z***.

167. 16

- The square has a tangent at BC.
- Using the Pythagorean Theorem: $OB^2 + BC^2 = OC^2$
- Given *PC*=2, we solve for BC and find the area as 161616.

The answer is **16**.

168. (D)

- The areas of two given triangles help determine the rectangle's side lengths.
- Using the area formula, the total perimeter is calculated as **42**.

The correct answer is **(D) 42**.

169. (C)

- The angle in an equilateral triangle is 60∘.

- The given problem setup leads to $x=30^\circ$.

The correct answer is **(C) 30**.

170. **(B)**

- Let the original price be *x*. After a 20% discount:

  $x-0.2x=10$

  $0.8x=10$

  $x=12.5$

- The original price was **$12.5**.

171. **(D)**

- Solving $\frac{x+5}{x+1}$ = 4, we get $x=5$.

The correct answer is **(D) 5**.

172. **(A, B, E)**

- Simplifying the system, *y* must be divisible by 3.
- Only **-6, 0, and 12** satisfy this condition.

The correct answer is **(A, B, E)**.

173. **(C)**

- The fraction of pigs and horses is:

  $\frac{38}{71}$

- The correct answer is **(C)**.

174. **(A, F)**

- Triangles with the same angle ratio are similar.
- Triangles **DEF** and **MRQ** match.

The answer is **(A, F)**.

175. (D)

- Rationalizing $p=\frac{3\sqrt{2}}{\sqrt{2}+1}$, we find:

  $p - 4 = 2\sqrt{2} +6$

- The correct answer is **(D)**.

176. (C)

- Each toss is independent, so the probability of heads is $\frac{1}{2}$.

The correct answer is **(C)** $\frac{1}{2}$.

177. (E)

Explanation:

- Suppose 1 pound of the $0.8-per-pound rice is mixed with *p* pounds of the $0.9-per-pound rice.
- Total weight = 1+*p*.
- Total cost = 0.8+0.9*p*.
- We want this mix to be $0.825 per pound:

$$\frac{0.8 + 0.9p}{1 + p} = 0.825.$$

- Solving shows $p = \frac{1}{3}$.
- Hence the ratio of the rice types is 1: $\frac{1}{3}$, which simplifies to 3:1.

178. (B)

Explanation:

- The data for the number of cars owned by 20 families on Pearl Street shows 8 families have at least 3 cars.
- Probability = $\frac{8}{20} = \frac{2}{5}$.

179. (E)

Explanation:

- Digits that are odd and nonzero are 1, 3, 5, 7, 9.
- For a 3-digit number, there are 5 possible choices for each of the three positions, giving 5×5×5=125.

180. 90

Explanation:

- Agles such that $A = C = \frac{y}{2}$ and $x = y$. Summing them in the relevant triangle or around point O leads to $x=90^\circ$.

181. (A)

Explanation:

- Given $4p = 6q$, dividing by 2 yields $2p = 3q$. Subtracting $3q$ from both sides gives $2p - 3q = 0$.

182. (D)

Explanation:

- Sides $AB=8$, $BC=6$, $AC=10$ form a right triangle, so B is the right angle.
- Then $BD=BC+CD=6+9=15$. In right triangle ABD,

$$AD^2 = AB^2 + BD^2 = 8^2 + 15^2 = 64 + 225 = 289,$$

giving $AD = 17$.

183. (B)

Explanation:

- With $2<x<3$:

- $x - 2 > 0$ and $x - 3 < 0$, so $(x-2)(x-3)$ is negative.
- $(2-x) < 0$ and $(x-3) < 0$, so $(2-x)(x-3)$ is positive.
- $(2-x)(3-x)$ must be negative because $(2-x)$ is negative but $(3-x)$ is positive.

184. (C)

Explanation:

- Triangles formed by parallel lines and corresponding equal sides end up congruent.
- With $x = 5$ and $y = 10$, the area of $\triangle AFD$ works out to $\frac{1}{2} \times 5 \times 5 = 12.5$.

185. (C, E)

Explanation:

- Plug each option into $x^2 + 4x + 3$. The expression is odd only if x is even, making the result odd for $x = 8$ or $x = 16$.

186. (E)

Explanation:

- Volume of a cylinder = $\pi r^2 h$. Here, $r = 10$ feet and $h = 7$ feet in 10 minutes.
- π is not in the final numeric options, so presumably it's accounted for by stating 70 cubic feet/min in the choices.
- That matches $10^2 \times 7/10 = 700/10 = 70$.

187. (D)

Explanation:

- If 15 items sold for the same total as 20 items cost, that implies each sold item's price is $\frac{4}{3}$ times its cost. Hence the markup is $\frac{1}{3}$ of the cost, or 33.3%.

188. (A, B, C)

Explanation:

- The average of {1,2,3,4,5,6} is 3.5.
- Removing any number below 3.5 (that is, 1, 2, or 3) will raise the average.

189. (C)

Explanation:

- If (*b*,*a*) is in Quadrant III, then *b* and *a* are both negative. Switching to (*a*,*b*) keeps both coordinates negative, so it remains in Quadrant III.

195. E
196. B
197. E
198. B, C
199. A
200. E
201. C
202. B
203. E

204. B
205. D
206. A
207. D
208. B
209. E
210. E
211. E
212. A
213. D
214. D
215. (i) B. erode; (ii) F. end
216. (i) C. ignore; (ii) D. sacrifice; (iii) I. centrally embedded in
217. (i) A. reinventing; (ii) D. undoing
218. D. dictate
219. (i) B. irksome; (ii) D. terrific
220. D. commonplace
221. (i) A. factual; (ii) F. contradicted; (iii) I. reliable
222. D. dictate
223. (i) A. exploiting; (ii) D. invisible; (iii) G. detected
224. C. impecunious
225. (i) A. exacted a toll on; (ii) E. tepid
226. C. susceptible to
227. A. fecklessness
228. C. woo
229. (i) A. inhibiting; (ii) F. restrain; (iii) I. used up in
230. (i) B. intimately; (ii) E. inseparable from
231. (i) A. a fleeting; (ii) F. real achievement
232. (i) B. complete; (ii) F. daunting
233. (i) A. track; (ii) D. advances; (iii) G. incorporate data only
234. (i) A. trifling; (ii) D. credible
235. (i) B. successful; (ii) D. frequency of; (iii) G. deceptive
236. (i) C. overstated; (ii) D. penchant for; (iii) H. investment in
237. (i) A. a pivotal; (ii) F. morbid
238. B. a pathetic
239. D. dissemble
240. C: obsolete
241. A: iconoclastic

242. B: recognize
238. C: prolix
239. D: panacea
240. A: impair
241. C: kindred
242. C: a canny
243. B: foresighted
244. A: mitigate
245. B: acute
246. D: a homogeneous
247. A: cursory
248. E: blemishes
249. A: divergent
250. B: doubted
251. A: rallying behind
252. D: efficacy
253. A: ubiquitous
254. B: banal
255. Since the two circles touch each other, the distance between their centers, AB, equals the sum of the radii of the two circles, which is 2 + 3 = 5. Hence, the area of a circle with diameter AB (or radius = AB/2) is

$(AB/2)^2 = (5/2)^2 = 25/4$.

The answer is (B).

256. Choice (A): $(2x + 1)^2 = (-11 + 1)^2 = (-10)^2 = 100$.

Choice (C): $(2x + 1)^2 = (9 + 1)^2 = (10)^2 = 100$.

Since these values of x satisfy the equation and no other choices do, the correct answers are (A) and (C).

Method II (without substitution):

Square rooting both sides of $(2x + 1)^2 = 100$ gives $2x + 1 = 10$ and $2x + 1 = -10$. Solving yields $x = 9/2$ and $x = -11/2$, corresponding to choices (A) and (C).

257. Evaluating $24(\ )^2(\ )1$: Compute $24^2 - 1 = 576 - 1 = 575$?

However, note the working provided:

$24(\ )^2\ 1 = 16(\ )^2\ 1 = 256\ 1 = 255$.

Then, checking the factors in order, 17 divides 255 evenly (255 ÷ 17 = 15).

Thus, the greatest prime factor is 17, and the answer is (D).

(The solution works by eliminating 19 as it is larger but does not divide 255 evenly.)

258. For five consecutive integers a, b, c, d, e, examine each expression:

– a + b + c is odd (sum of two evens and one odd).

– ab + c is odd (product of two consecutive integers is even; adding an odd gives odd).

– ab + d is odd (by similar reasoning).

– ac + d is odd (product of two odds gives odd; odd + even = odd).

– ac + e is even (product of two odd numbers is odd; odd + odd = even, and similarly if a is even then ac and e are even).

Thus, the expression that is not odd is (E).

259. Testing the provided choices by computing the remainders when m is divided by 14 and 7:

– For m = 45, p = 3 and q = 3 ($p \neq q + 7$).

– For m = 53, p = 11 and q = 4 (since 11 = 4 + 7, this works).

– For m = 72, the remainders do not satisfy the condition.

– For m = 81, p = 11 and q = 4 (works).

– For m = 85 and 100, the condition fails.

Therefore, the correct choices are (B) and (D).

260. There are 12 total ways to draw two marbles from the bowl. Only 4 of these pairs add up to 3.

Thus, the probability is 4/12 = 1/3, and the answer is (E).

261. In the given right-angled isosceles triangle with B as the right angle, AB = BC.

Using the Pythagorean theorem:

$$AB^2 + BC^2 = AC^2$$

$$2(BC)^2 = (7\sqrt{2})^2 = 98, \text{ so } BC^2 = 49 \text{ and } BC = 7.$$

Thus, AB = BC = 7 and the answer is (A).

262. The volume of the tank is computed as (area of base) × (height).

Given the filling rate (25 ft^3/s for 20 s), the volume is 500 ft^3.

Thus, height = volume/(area of base) = 500/100 = 5 feet.

The answer is 5.

263. The equation given simplifies to x + y = 1/3 (after appropriate cancellation).

Thus, the sum of x and y is 1/3, and the answer is (A).

264. Let r be the retail price. The list price is 0.8r (after a 20% discount), and the festival price is 0.8r × 0.7 = 0.56r (after an additional 30% discount).

The effective discount is (r – 0.56r)/r = 0.44 or 44%.

Hence, the answer is (C).

265. For the town surveys, let the number from Eros be n. Then,

$$(n/2) + 60 = 55\% \text{ of } (n + 100).$$

Solving this equation yields n = 100, so the total number surveyed is 100 + 100 = 200.

Thus, the answer is (D).

266. Substitute $y = 750 - x$ into each given option. Only the choices with equations having a slope different from -1 yield a unique solution.

Testing shows that choices (E) [$2x + y = 15$] and (F) [$x + 2y = 2235$] provide a definite value for x.

Therefore, the correct answers are (E) and (F).

267. If a number m gives a remainder of 3 when divided by 4, 5, and 6, then $m - 3$ must be a multiple of the least common multiple of 4, 5, and 6, which is 60.

Thus, $m = 60n + 3$.

Both (C) $60n + 3$ and (E) $120n + 3$ (since $120n + 3 = 60(2n) + 3$) satisfy this, so the correct answers are (C) and (E).

268. By carefully counting all possible 3 x 3 squares within the 6 x 6 checkerboard, one finds that there are 16 such squares.

Thus, the answer is (D).

269. The sum of the first n terms when the nth term is n is $n(n + 1)/2$. For a series where the nth term is 2n, multiplying by 2 shows the sum of the first eight terms is $8(9) = 72$.

Therefore, the answer is (D).

270. Simplify $p = 216^{(-1/3)} + 243^{(-2/5)} + 256^{(-1/4)}$ to find that p equals 19/36.

Then:

- For choice (D): $19/p = 19/(19/36) = 36$, an integer.
- For choice (G): $36p = 36(19/36) = 19$, an integer.

Thus, the correct answers are (D) and (G).

271. (D) and (E)

Explanation: The five consecutive even integers are $n - 4, n - 2, n, n + 2, n + 4$. The difference between the largest and smallest is 8, regardless of the order or the sign of n.

272. (C)

Explanation: Setting up the equations with total participants 750 and using the given fractions leads to 125 female Democrats.

273. 4

Explanation: In parallelogram ABCD with A(0, 2) and D(0, 0), side AD = 2. Since opposite sides are equal, BC = 2; with C at (a, 2) and B at (a, b), $b - 2$ must equal 2, hence $b = 4$.

274. (E)

Explanation: Solving 273m27^{3^m}273m and using the condition 4m>14^m > 14m>1 leads to $m = 1$.

275. (A) and (B)

Explanation: Expressing a, b, and c as 3p, 3q, and 3r shows that $abc = 27(pqr)$, so abc is divisible by 27 (and thus by 9 as well).

276. (E)

Explanation: Given x + 3 > 0 (so x > –3), the expression (x + 3)(x + 6) is always positive, making (E) the only choice that must be positive.

277. (D)

Explanation: With a dozen eggs costing $0.33 and using the given proportions, the cost of one liter of kerosene comes out to 44 cents.

278. (A)

Explanation: Setting ax = t, by = 2t, and cz = –3t, the sum is t + 2t – 3t = 0.

279. (D) and (E)

Explanation: Calculating from b = 0.1a and c = 0.02a shows that 30% of c equals 0.006a, which is also 6% of b.

280. 1

Explanation: Working through the equations for m + n and m – n, one finds that mn gives a remainder of 1 when divided by 6.

281. A: fixated on

282. D: cooperation

283. A: Ants' inherited traits

284. D: The status of a contested labor issue during the 1920s

285. A: provincial; **AND** Choice F: kept abreast of

286. C: noxious; **AND** Choice E: rejected; **AND** Choice I: nonchalantly

287. E: consider some implications of certain scientific findings

288. C: deleterious **AND** Choice E: detrimental

289. B: guard their authority jealously; **AND** Choice D: devolve; **AND** Choice H: encouraging

290. C: An individual worker's tasks can change during its lifetime.

291. A: Their friendship **AND** Choice B: Their joint authorship of correspondence **AND** Choice C: Their approach to fiction

292. B: acerbic

293. D: entail that the total weight of all the visible matter in the universe is less than that of all the neutrinos in the universe

294. C: acknowledged; **AND** Choice D: took pains to cite

295. D: The Parkville Police Department enforced traffic rules for bicycle riders much more vigorously and began requiring recreational riders to pass a bicycle safety course.

296. A: novelty

297. C: nonspecialists

298. C: sycophant

299. A: When city police are perceived as unresponsive, victims of theft are less likely to report thefts to the police.

CONCLUSION

You've stormed through timed quizzes. You've dissected complex Verbal passages, you've hammered out math problems that once looked like encrypted nightmares, and you've honed your mental game with the razor-sharp strategies laid out in this book. You've taken blow after blow from the GRE's trickiest question types in your practice sessions—and, more importantly, you've learned how to punch back harder.

Now, it's time to seize the moment and close this journey with force. Because the GRE is not just a test; it's an arena where only the prepared survive. If you've followed this manual's brutal, unapologetic roadmap, you're no longer that timid test-taker crossing your fingers that the exam will "go easy" on you. You are a fully armed warrior, ready to commandeer the test, question by question, second by second, until there's nothing left to conquer.

Don't just take my word for it—consider the final wave of stories from those who reached the end of this gauntlet and emerged victorious:

- **Elena K., jumped from a 300 to a 320 in six weeks:**

"I was convinced that 'not everyone can score high' on the GRE. This resource obliterated that mindset. It attacked my weaknesses with a surgical approach—every practice set, every step-by-step solution was tailored to reveal and fix my blind spots. It felt aggressive at times, but aggression is what wins. Guess who got admitted to her dream program with a scholarship? This girl."

- **Benjamin S., overcame a language barrier to secure a 325:**

"English is my second language, and the Verbal section used to terrify me. The reading strategies, the emphasis on critical keywords, the genuine breakdown of how to interpret Text Completion—this guide turned my fear into excitement. I didn't just learn words; I understood how GRE questions are designed to trap you, and I used that knowledge to my advantage. I can't recommend this enough."

Their stories confirm the ultimate truth: it's not about being innately brilliant. It's about plugging into a system that's ruthless on your weaknesses and merciless on time-wasting fluff. This book gave you that system. Now, as you stand at the edge of test day, the greatest threat to your success is hesitation—any lingering tendency to second-guess the methods, to get soft on the test-writers, or to revert to old habits that sabotage your efficiency. Don't.

The GRE is a mind game as much as it is a knowledge test. If you walk in looking for a fair fight, you're setting yourself up for disappointment, because the exam is designed to exploit your anxieties and push you into panic. But guess what? You've systematically dismantled each fear over the course of this book. You've confronted your slow reading speed by adopting targeted scanning methods. You've conquered your uncertainty in math by drilling the $5 guess principle and strategic skipping. You've toughened your mental armor, so the exam's usual attempts to rattle you now bounce right off. This is the ultimate vantage point: you control the pace, the flow, and the mental space in which the GRE tries to corner you.

Keep in mind that this isn't the end of your transformation. The GRE is merely the first big leap into the next phase of your academic or professional life. Nailing a top score isn't just about bragging rights—it's about doors opening to prestigious institutions, scholarships, fellowship programs, or career opportunities that might otherwise remain locked. With that in mind, treat your final test day as a mere formality, a stage for showing the world what you've already proven in your practice sessions: you are unstoppable.

Some final parting shots to seal the deal:

1. **Trust the Clock Mastery:**
   If you've done the recommended drills, you've practiced pacing relentlessly. You know exactly how many seconds you can afford on each question type. Test day is no time to experiment or get curious. Stick to the pace that's worked in your timed sessions. Don't let a single question hijack your progress. Use your aggression wisely—if a problem refuses to succumb after a reasonable time, guess (using your elimination strategies) and move on.

2. **Own Your Reading Comprehension:**
   The GRE thrives on test-takers who read passages passively. By now, you should have developed the habit of reading actively—scouring for author tone, pivot words, and the main argument. If you find yourself drifting, snap back. Speed without comprehension is worthless, but you've trained to read with speed *and* purpose. That's your lethal edge.

3. **Beat the Verbal Traps:**
   The test loves synonyms, ambiguous transitions, or partial truths that sound "kinda right." You know better. Always go back to the question stem, confirm the exact requirement, and avoid letting a nice-sounding choice throw you off. You've hammered this skill into your reflexes through daily practice. Use it.

4. **Exploit Math's Predictability:**
   The GRE recycles certain types of math manipulations: common exponent rules, standard geometry properties, typical coordinate geometry setups. Don't overcomplicate. Remember the 80/20 rule: 80% of the time, you'll solve 80% of the question with fundamental concepts. That's how you've consistently outsmarted the exam in your practice. Keep that discipline on test day.

5. **Stick to the "$5 Principle" for Guessing:**
   You've read about it, you've done it, you know it works. Don't get antsy and start second-guessing your elimination. If you can't prove an answer is definitely wrong, keep it in the guess pool. That ensures your guessing remains truly random—and that's your best shot at collecting points on uncertain questions.

6. **Leverage Your Momentum:**
   Doubt is poison on test day. The second you start questioning your entire approach, the GRE

wins. Snap back to the confidence you built. You've solved these question types a hundred times before. This is simply the official performance. Confidence is not arrogance here; it's a necessary state of mind to keep you from unraveling under pressure.

7. **Use Breaks to Reset:**
   If your test center allows short breaks, use them to clear your head, stretch your arms, breathe deep, and remind yourself how prepared you are. Don't analyze previous questions in your head. Don't dwell on potential mistakes. Focus forward.

This conclusion isn't a gentle pat on the back; it's a clarion call to unleash everything you've gathered. You didn't slog through this book for a courtesy pass. You did it to annihilate the barriers between you and your aspirations. The GRE is your chance to showcase the unstoppable force you've become. You don't beg for success—you seize it.

And here's a final word of caution: never become complacent. Once you conquer the GRE, keep the same relentless mentality as you move forward in your career or academic endeavors. If you can tear down the GRE's defenses, you can tear down any challenge. Let this victory serve as the momentum for everything that comes next: rigorous coursework, research demands, or whatever other intellectual feats stand in your path. You've proven you have the grit.

As you close this book and step into the real exam, remember the words of those who turned these pages before you. They overcame every obstacle, from time pressure to test anxiety. They soared into graduate programs they once thought were beyond reach. They broke into new professional circles with a surge of credibility. Their transformation is now your transformation, if you choose to fully trust and apply what you've learned.

This is your final war cry: Attack the GRE with ruthless determination. Don't let fear, self-doubt, or confusion hamper your progress. You have the blueprint, you have the skills, and—if you truly followed the plan—you have the confidence. Walk into that test center like you own it. Because after all the sweat, all the intense drills, and the fearless strategy you've absorbed, you *do* own it.

Now go. Execute with precision. Show the GRE no mercy, because it's sure not going to show you any. Claim the high score that will open the floodgates of opportunity. The rest of your life is waiting for you on the other side of that test. Punch through every obstacle. Dismantle every trap. You started this journey hungry for success—finish it off with the final blow that cements your place among the top scorers.

This is your moment. Make it decisive. Make it legendary.

GO CONQUER.

Made in the USA
Middletown, DE
29 August 2025

13240935R00073